Pietà

Pietà

George Klein

translated by Theodore and Ingrid Friedmann

The MIT Press
Cambridge, Massachusetts
London, England

First MIT Press edition
English translation © 1992 Massachusetts Institute of Technology

© 1989 George Klein. First published, in Swedish, as *Pietà* (Stockholm: Albert
Bonniers Förlag AB).

This book was set in New Baskerville by The MIT Press and was printed and
bound in the United States of America.

Library of Congress Cataloging-in-Publication Data

Klein, George, 1925–
    [Pietà. English]
    Pietà / George Klein ; translated by Theodore and Ingrid Friedmann.
      p. cm.
    Includes bibliographical references (p.   ) and index.
    ISBN 0-262-11161-6
    1. Life.   2. Suffering.   I. Title.
BD435.K48413   1992
128—dc20
                                                      92-18900
                                                        CIP

To the memory of Kaszony, my father's village—gone forever but ever present, more powerful than the smells and tastes of the past, warmer than love and, unlike pain, unfading.

Contents

Preface

No two human beings have exactly the same fingerprints or the same tissue proteins, except in the case of identical twins. Nor are there any two authors who use the same methods for writing a book.

Some are secretive—no one is allowed to know anything of their work until the book is finished. Others show little bits and pieces to their intimate friends as a symbol of their confidence.

I don't belong to either of these categories. I feel like a small child about to take his first step. I wonder, is the degree of insecurity greater if one doesn't learn to walk until late? Or does it represent damage sustained over many years of scientific writing, in which one is always concerned about the comments of colleagues, even though the literary quality of scientific papers is taken about as seriously as the libretto of a bel canto opera.

Whatever the case, this book, like my previous books, would not have been possible without the help of many good friends. They have reacted, criticized, commented, and edited the Swedish original, with unending interest. I want to thank Per Ahlmark, Heinrich Artmann, Benkt Erik Benktsson, Tore Browaldh, Peter Citron, Lone Dueholm, Egon Fenyö, Karl-Erik Fichtelius, Kerstin Fredga, Inga Gottfarb, Lars Gyllensten, Ulf Lagerkvist, Göran Larsson, Rolf Luft, Tryggve Mettinger, Benno Müller-Hill, Anders Nässil, Lennart Philipson, Mark Ptashne, Dagmar Reichard, Geza Thinsz, Per Uddén, Lars Ulvenstam, Hans Wigzell, and Per Wästberg for their invaluable help.

I also want to thank my secretaries, none of them named but none forgotten, for their typing and revising and for their discreet but necessary correction of my words. Without the help of Karin Jacobsson, this book would never have come into being. And my wife Eva had only to blink her eyes or wrinkle her forehead.

Pietà

Part One

1

Introduction

There is but one truly philosophical problem, and that is suicide. Judging whether life is or is not worth living amounts to answering the fundamental question of philosophy.

Albert Camus, *The Myth of Sisyphus*[1]

The problem posed by Camus is as old as humanity, but its relevance and interest never diminish. We all know about it, whether or not we choose to acknowledge it. It is with the same equanimity that we look, in art museums, upon the rapt faces expressing an artist's vision of divine delight and the horrifying demons of Hieronymus Bosch's paintings. The snow-white wings of Psyche and the thousand venomous heads of the hydra exist side by side in our soul. Like Dante, we go astray constantly in the *selva oscura* of our lives, the forest where darkness, the only true democrat, awaits men and women, rich and poor, beautiful and ugly, sophisticated and simple, with the same complete indifference.

Some find their Virgil, their teacher and guide. Beatrice remembers some lost souls in her paradise. A persevering ascent to the starlit summit, with the weight on the lower foot, can save some of these souls, at least for the moment. But all solutions are transient; the dilemma remains, whether one chooses not to discuss it or to talk about it incessantly. Faust's last word before he drinks the poisoned wine, the very first word in Gounod's operatic version of the legend, is *Rien!* (Nothing!). It is a word that recurs every day in billions of versions. It is sung by the pop group The Fugs in their pulsating, captivating song "Nothing," which condemns everything and everyone. It lives and dies with young drug addicts; it is shrieked to deaf ears by the outcasts; it is concealed, camouflaged, and distorted beyond recognition by those who have "succeeded." The Faust legend is with us forever, although Mephistopheles has vanished, at least as a romantic figure in his enchanting red costume. A soul that is not eternal can no longer be sold for the reward of pleasure and oblivion. Mephistopheles was able to help Faust only temporarily, despite the fact that Faust signed the contract in blood. This is the inevitable moral conclusion of the legend. The "golden tree" of life could not mitigate Faust's collision with his sense of meaninglessness following his lifelong search through the world of human knowledge.

Why have those who have chosen suicide answered no to the fundamental philosophical question posed by Camus? Were they courageous or cowardly? Did they act of their free will and with moral consistency, as did Seneca and Socrates, or did they follow a sudden impulse of desperation? We all follow different paths, whether they lead up or down. Among the vast numbers of suicide victims, whom the living find so puzzling, one can easily find both kinds. One who planned well was Arthur Koestler, who left us— after a life of occasionally well-reasoned but more often loose, albeit brilliant, speculations about the human condition—together with his young wife Cynthia, in a final majestic performance. I also recall the example of the dean of French cancer researchers, Professor Lacassagne, who worked until the day before his death in his eighties. He lived on the top floor of an old and fashionable apartment house in Paris. On his last morning his maid, dressed in her black and white uniform and lace cap, served him his coffee as usual. It was a long and uninterrupted tradition. The coffee was particularly delicious that day. The professor praised it, asked for another cup, and then jumped out of the window. What thoughts could he have had before he jumped? Was he aware of what he was about to do, or did he surrender to a sudden feeling of despair?

Another colleague of mine telephoned the administrative offices at the university to ask about the pension and social benefits his family would receive if he happened to die. The people at the office thought he was inquiring because he had questions about an insurance policy, and they told him that they would work out the terms of the pension for him. Two weeks later, they telephoned and told him what they had found out. "Thank you very much," said the professor. He hung up and shot himself. I've always wondered what he would have done if the amount of his pension had been smaller. Would he have hesitated, like so many others who have responded negatively to Camus's philosophical question, but refrained from carrying it to its ultimate conclusion?

Shakespeare's Hamlet is the most famous of those who have hesitated. In his famous soliloquy, he examines the question of whether life is worth living, and reaches a basically negative conclusion:

For who would bear the whips and scorns of time,
The oppressor's wrong, the proud man's contumely,
The pangs of disprized love, the law's delay,
The insolence of office, and the spurns
That patient merit of the unworthy takes,
When he himself might his quietus make
With a bare bodkin?

But Hamlet feared the dreams that might come in that sleep of death, of which no one knew anything. He hesitated. His depression reflects one aspect of reality, as was true of Faust, but it excludes another. It is somewhat like looking at the drawings of Escher, in which black birds are flying to the right while white ones are going to the left. It is not possible to visualize both at the same time. As long as one concentrates on the black birds, one cannot see the white ones. Hamlet could not see the white bird, the will to live. Faust could see it for only a short time, and then only with the help of Mephistopheles.

Some of us are able to see the white birds more easily than the black ones, whereas for others it is quite the opposite. Is it possible to train oneself to switch from the black to the white, or is that possible only for those who, for some reason, are predestined not to answer no to Camus's question?

Anxiety over this question is one of the principal colored strands woven through the fabric of this book. I have tried to study some who managed to lift themselves out of the darkness, and others who succumbed. I have tried to write about their lives and their deaths. I would have liked to look out from atop their shoulders, to place my ears to their heads and sense their struggle to reach the light. I also wanted to follow them down the road of their despair, to the end and to the darkness. But no one can climb inside another person—for each of us, only our subjective world exists. We do not know what occurs in the soul of another human being, only what transpires within ourselves. Nevertheless, I have tried. Superficially and haltingly, with language as my only instrument, with stumbling and stammering, I have tried to approach some whose path has led downward. One was a very close relative who could have become a great poet if he hadn't taken his own life at the age of eighteen. The other, Attila József, was a great poet, one of the greatest in the rich history of Hungarian poetry. He tried to commit suicide during his teens, and finally succeeded at the age of thirty-two. During his short life he became the "educator of the entire nation" and the "surveyor of the human condition." He was able to "edit the inner harmony . . . enable his mind to perceive the limited eternity, the creative external forces and internal drives." Those who read his works today, more than half a century after his death, have the same experience. But even his extraordinary talent could not save him. Is there any hope of understanding, or at least anticipating, why the idolized poet of an entire nation preferred the steely, silent, and unmerciful wheels of a train?

Many poets have described the black bird of depression, the specter that paralyzes the soul. Of the relatively few poets with whom I am familiar, none has accomplished it with the same immense power and enchanting beauty as Edgar Allan Poe. I beg the forgiveness of the reader when I take off my hat, step aside, and let the poet speak for himself for a while. Poe maintains that he wrote his poems with cold calculation, trying simply to impress the reader. And yet, if that were the case, why did he die in a fit of delerium tremens, after he had forced the entire literary world to its knees time and again?

To what extent can creative activity help? Which of us can rise up out of the swamp of his own soul, to transform the deadly trap into an unending source of inspiration? How are some able to convert explosives into fuel to drive the subtle and fragile machinery of their talents? How can they build up their inner strength and use it to turn their personal demons into constructive and obedient little helpers, who can support their creative activity without interruption? It is not only the process of creativity that is driven by these tamed furies, but also the ability of the creative machinery to reach others. They are the source of the machinery; they are simultaneously the tightrope walker's wire and the abyss underneath. They are the volcanic crater and the narrow path along its rim where one can leisurely stroll. Is it just random chance that determines who falls at an early stage, who leaps willingly to end the tragedy, and who balances on the razor-sharp edge until the very end? How important are the impulses from within, the will to win, the power of defiance? One of the greatest winners, Thomas Mann, said that creativity succeeds "in spite of" rather than "because of." Rainer Maria Rilke, another master in the same category, to whom I must always return, said, "I sense that I can, I seize the day and shape it."

"*A te convien tenere altro viaggio*" — "You must choose another path," Virgil tells Dante before leading him out of the dark forest.[2] But which path did he originally wish to follow before he abandoned the "true path" (*verace via*) during a trancelike walk (*pien di sonno*) in "the middle of our life's journey?" Where will he arrive with Virgil's help—with the help of poetry? Before Virgil arrived, all exits were closed. He tried to climb to the summit of the mountain, to "see the stars once again," but three wild beasts blocked his way—the lion, representing haughtiness and ambition, the symbol of the French kingdom; the panther, representing lust, Dante's image of artistic and degenerate Florence; and the greedy she-wolf, always in heat, representing the insatiable thirst of the papacy for worldly power and possessions.

The stars (*le stelle*) is a frequently used term in *The Divine Comedy*. Beatrice's eyes "surpassed the splendor of the stars" (*lucevan gli occhi suoi più che la stella*) when she visited Virgil to express her compassion with the poet gone astray. All three parts of the *Divine Comedy* —*Inferno*, *Purgatory*, and *Paradise*—close with the same word. Dante and Virgil emerge through a narrow tunnel from the deepest abyss of hell through a narrow tunnel, and at the opening they "can see the stars again" (*a riveder le stelle*). When Dante reaches the top of the mountain in *Purgatory*, he feels pure and, together with Beatrice, is prepared to ascend to the stars (*puro e disposto a salire alle stelle*). The final divine vision in *Paradise* is a revelation of "the love that moves the sun and the other stars" (*l'amor che move il sole e l'altre stelle*).[3]

In *The Divine Comedy*, Dante was led from the dark forest to the redeeming encounter with his own soul by the sublimation of religion, the universal wishful thinking that was still widely perceived as reality. But we would never have heard of Dante if he hadn't been driven by his incomparably poetic inspiration, which he modestly attributed to the master Virgil. Whoever wishes to give himself a lifelong gift should follow Dante through the bustling world of the Renaissance as described in the hundred cantos of this immortal work, a divine comedy indeed. Its theological burden, out of date as it is, is as light as a feather compared with the timeless description of the human condition. A contemporary reader following a path through this masterpiece for possibly the tenth time—who knows what obstacles to avoid—perks up and pays attention whenever he encounters the word "like" (*come*), which signals a metaphor describing anguish, despair, or the fragile bloom of hope. The pilgrim Dante feels like a shipwreck survivor who reaches shore and looks back, exhausted and gasping, at the raging sea (see *Inferno*, Canto 1, sentence 22), or like a gambler who anxiously guards his winnings but who decries his lust for gambling when he loses (I: 56). Like the doubts that devour the first impulse, the plan blocked by new plans (II: 37), the beast frightened by its own dreams (II: 48), a frozen flower, shut and bent by the chill of the night, when it rises up and opens fully in the sunshine (II: 127), the damned souls attracted by a soothing word, like the dove flying toward its soft nest (V: 82). The experienced reader, walking along this path, will find himself in the present day—he will find you and me, our common experience. One is no longer alone: Dante had the same feelings, and millions more must feel the same way every day.

What was the most essential element in the development of Dante's own astounding inner sources of power? Was it his ability to resist the temptations symbolized by the beasts, or to defy his exile from Florence, to which he responded with the thundering two words *nunquam revertar* —I shall never return? Was it his ability to endure all disappointments and treacheries? Was it Beatrice, the personification of all undelivered desires and aspirations? Was it the dream about the blessed woman who cares for her friend gone astray? Or was it first and foremost his own sense of creativity, the "lovely style that has brought honor to me," the immense power of his language, life transformed into poetry to protect from life?

Dante, Rilke, Poe, Baudelaire, Attila József, and a few other poets have often been of great sustenance to me. They have succeeded in expressing a true or imaginary experience—the experience of suffering—with such acuity and remarkable originality that I have often been forced to listen with rapt attention and forget my own troubles. I assume that they have sustained many others in the same way, otherwise their work would not have survived. The survival of their work is probably due to their ability to convey the universality of suffering and allow it to penetrate the barriers of differences in history, culture, and language. The vital significance of this became particularly clear to me during the fateful year 1944, when 80 percent of us Hungarian Jews were being gassed, starved, beaten to death, or in some other way murdered. There are some occasions, some life-threatening situations, in which one's willpower and courage are tested to the extreme. These are times when particular combinations of words, words of a great poet, flow up from the subconscious and give us the strength to resist the opposing urge—buried deeply but always ready to appear—to follow the path of least resistance (even if it means going like cattle to the slaughterhouse), to escape the responsibility of thinking and acting. I do not believe that I am unique in assigning such power to ingeniously phrased words. I have heard similar stories from other survivors from varied backgrounds. Consider, for instance, the line from Dante that I have chosen as the motif for the chapter "The Ultimate Fear of the Traveler Returning from Hell": ". . . . *Tant' è amara che poco è più morte*" (so bitter death is hardly more severe).

At first, I was probably merely attracted by the perfect form and sound of that line. But suddenly, when I began interpreting the meaning of those words for myself, to taste them and feel them inside me, they took on a new meaning that is not necessarily the same as that intended by the poet. What is so bitter that death can hardly surpass it, if not life itself—life as described in Dante's *Inferno*, a visionary and often highly theological but accurate portrayal of suffering, then and now. Dante does not have to endure all the hellish torments himself to have a clear insight into what they are truly like. It is sufficient for him to encounter the condemned souls and hear their tales. His empathy for their suffering is so deep that his own life seems to escape from him (*cos'io morisse*) and he faints or, in his words, falls "as a dead body falls" (*e caddi come corpo morto cade*).

Death may be only slightly more burdensome than life. It may even be less burdensome. That knowledge can be transformed into a bright ray of hope—but not the religious or illusory hope for human goodness and a better world of an unrealistic utopia. On the contrary, the hope might be the knowledge that all suffering, even the most extreme, will have an end.

Very few writers have the ability to express the reality of suffering in poetry whose music and wordcraft forces the reader to lift his head and listen intently, shutting out the teeming world with its thousands of distractions. Most people cannot describe their suffering well enough to induce the empathy of the reader. I have talked with many "travelers through hell," survivors of the concentration camps and other who have come close to apocalyptic experiences and have been unable to express their torment in words. Their inability to describe the journey through hell in a language understood by others makes it impossible for them to either help others or rescue themselves. Many remain completely silent, others are ashamed of what they have endured. Why ashamed? Do they come to accept the label given them by the executioner? Are they filled with unending and incurable rage?

The poet who most successfully gave literary expression to the undescribable was Paul Celan, who in the end took his own life. His poem "Death Fugue" (*Todesfuge*) is one long sentence. Here is one small part of it:

Schwarze Milch der Frühe wir trinken sie abends
wir trinken sie mittags und morgens wir trinken sie nachts
wir trinken und trinken
wir schaufeln ein Grab in den Lüften da liegt man nicht eng

Ein mann wohnt im Haus der spielt mit den Schlangen der schreibt
der schreibt wenn es dunkelt nach Deutschland dein goldenes Haar
    Margarete
er schreibt es und tritt vor das Haus und es blitzen die Sterne er
    pfeift seine Rüden herbei
er pfeift seine Juden hervor lässt schaufeln ein Grab in der Erde

Er ruft spielt süsser den Tod Der Tod ist ein Meister aus
    Deutschland
er ruft streicht dunkler die Geigen dann steigt ihr als Rauch in die
    Luft
dan habt ihr ein Grab in den Wolken da liegt man nicht eng
Schwarze Milch der Frühe wir trinken dich nachts
wir trinken dich mittags der Tod ist ein Meister aus Deutschland
wir trinken dich abends und morgens wir trinken und trinken
der Tod ist ein Meister aus Deutschland sein Auge ist blau

er spielt mit den Schlangen und träumet der Tod ist ein Meister aus
    Deutschland
dein goldenes Haar Margarete
dein ashenes Haar Sulamith

Black milk of daybreak we drink it at sundown
we drink it at noon in the morning we drink it at night
we drink and we drink it
we dig a grave in the breezes there one lies unconfined
A man lives in the house he plays with the serpents he writes
he writes when dusk falls to Germany your golden hair
    Margarete
he writes it and steps out of doors and the stars are flashing he
    whistles his pack out
he whistles his Jews out in earth has them dig for a grave

He calls out more sweetly play death death is a master from
    Germany
he calls out more darkly now stroke your strings then as smoke
    you will rise into air
then a grave you will have in the clouds there one lies unconfined

Black milk of daybreak we drink you at night
we drink you at noon death is a master from Germany
we drink you at sundown and in the morning we drink and we
    drink you
death is a master from Germany his eyes are blue

he plays with the serpents and daydreams death is a master from
    Germany
your golden hair Margarete
your ashen hair Sulamith

Was it Auschwitz that finally caught up with Paul Celan when he took his own life? Is it true, as the psychologist Bruno Bettelheim hypothesized, that the death camps always catch up with their victims? Bettelheim was himself an inmate of a concentration camp early in the Nazi era, and recently he took his own life. Was it the same fate that befell the great prose writer of the holocaust, Primo Levi, whose voice, so unassuming and yet so profoundly incisive, gave such a convincing description of how it really was, and how vulnerable we all are to a similar fate? Despite the fact that Primo Levi was able to describe the experience of the infernal world of Auschwitz far more effectively than anyone else, he was thoroughly convinced that it was basically impossible to convey it to others. It is not only the lack of direct experience that makes most listeners unreceptive; there is also a natural reluctance to accept the idea that the fundamental psychological makeup of our species could be so evil.

Should such dark knowledge be divulged at all? Wouldn't it be better to protect our children from such unpleasant insights into human nature? If so, how are those who are so sheltered to react when they read about the most recent murders on the front page of the newspaper? Is it possible to throw this kind of information onto a refuse heap in the farthest recesses of the subconscious, label it "trash of no concern to me," and file it away? Should these violent criminals be locked away, provided that they can be found—should they be regarded as second-class citizens? Isn't it a bit too easy to slip from there into a kind of discrimination, to something dangerously close to racism? Shouldn't we first look into ourselves, to see the hidden violence deep in our soul, in the soul of our species? Of course, the outlaws among us must be held responsible for their deeds, but this century of Auschwitz and Hiroshima has made it impossible to maintain a clear-cut distinction between the blessed and the condemned. Purgatory is long gone, and Inferno and Paradise have been drawn together and their boundaries blurred. The experiences drawn from the mass murders and other monstrous crimes perpetrated by the Third Reich, the human experiments performed by the Japanese in Manchuria during the Second World War, and even the unethical experiments on unsuspecting volunteers supported by the CIA during the McCarthy era point toward one general conclusion:

crimes and mass murder sanctioned and perpetrated by a ruling power structure are only very rarely carried out directly by sadists and other psychopaths. Most of the perpetrators of such crimes and their bosses are merely the obedient and opportunistic servants of the system who consider their actions proper and lawful and who therefore have clear consciences. The SS physician Dr. Münch commented in an 1984 interview with Bernhard Frankfurther on Austrian television:

Everything at Auschwitz was programmed. Those serving there were all individually innocent and quite simple people who took refuge behind their pledges of loyalty and who imagined that they were only doing their duty. And they indeed did their duty in an especially commendable way, considering that they had such an extremely difficult assignment. I have spoken to many of them, both officers and ordinary soldiers, people whose hearts were not in sympathy with all that occurred at Auschwitz, but who did not imagine, even in conversations among friends, raising any objections or voicing any doubts whatsoever. It simply wasn't appropriate—and here I can find a certain rationale—it wasn't the thing to do. That's how it was, that was the way things were done, and that was just fine. Everything else was repressed and pushed aside.

The question of how such a system could come into being is interesting, but its minor, well-adjusted servants are not. Of special interest are those nonconformists with the courage and strength to follow their consciences and reject the spirit of the times, even if it meant enormous danger to them. Who were these people—what drove them? That question shatters into thousands of pieces as soon as one begins to examine it. In the essay on the fatherless, I have tried to look at this question from a very narrow perspective, as if through a keyhole. The absence of a father figure's superego, the inability to give or take orders without smiling, the inability to take hierarchical organizations and dignitaries seriously—these are factors that can contribute to the development of a nonconformist. But the lack of a father figure is not a decisive factor. There are many examples of nonconformists who have had good and strong relationships with their fathers. Nor is there any assurance, to use Sartre's words, that a "swimmer who does not have to carry his Anchises on his back" will always become a Raoul Wallenberg or a Franz Jägerstätter, rather than a terrorist or a bank robber.

What is this book all about? Suicide victims, the holocaust, poets?

No, I actually don't believe that the book is centered around any of these subjects. I have chosen them to help pose some questions regarding the human condition that seem essential to me. Poets—the "surveyors" of the human condition, as Attila József describes them—can understand its absurdities better than most others. The holocaust is the ultimate example of the evil within us. AIDS reminds us of unexpected dangers that lurk in the microbiological world around us, which can invade our seemingly well-protected existence at any time, when we least expect it. Our biological individuality remains one of the most powerful instruments for the survival of our species; it is one of the foundations of the enormous versatility of our immune defense system, the protective shield that defends our DNA from the threats of the microbiological world—a remarkable protection indeed, provided that our own brains do not endanger the same DNA with a nuclear war.

The victims of suicide, those who have rejected life—are they cowardly or are they brave? Do we despise or admire them? Are we fearful of them? All or none of the above?

I don't know. But I do know that the subjects I have been writing about have made me listen. They have forced their way into my conscience and at times have induced me "to play life itself in rapture,without thinking of approval" (. . .*hingerissen, das Leben spielen, nicht auf Beifall denkend*), just like the experiences with death described in Rilke's "Todeserfahrung."

But I know why the book has the title that it does. The unfathomable word *pietà* forces us to confront some of our most serious dilemmas. It is a word that no one has succeeded in translating into any other language—it loses all of its nuances in translation. Despite Schopenhauer's vast philological and literary knowledge and his philosophical and analytical acuity, he used the original Italian word when he chose to interpret the concept in his own special and obstinate way (see the chapter entitled "Pietà"). His interpretation of the word grew out of his concept of "blind will," the force that drives all living creatures and that may be compared, in modern terminology, with the intrinsic urge for replication of our "selfish genes" (see my essay on "Blind Will and Selfish DNA," in *The Atheist and the Holy City,* MIT Press, 1990). As conceived by Schopenhauer,[4] the will is fragmented into billions of individual creatures within each species, but that fragmentation does not diminish its power. The principle of individuation (*principium individuationis*) implies that each creature is driven by the will as if it were alone in the world. Schopenhauer writes:

Thus everywhere in nature we see strife, conflict and alternation of victory. . . . every grade of the objectification of will fights for the matter, the space, and the time of the others. . . . for each animal can only maintain its existence by the constant destruction of some other. Thus, the will to live everywhere preys upon itself, and in different forms is its own nourishment, till finally the human race. . . . because it subdues all the others, regards nature as a manufactory for its use. The fight that stems from the splitting of the will between different individuals manifests itself with its most terrible distinctness exactly in this species, so that human beings become like wolves toward each other, "*homo homini lupus*". . . .The will itself, the "thing-in-itself," is without ground. Therefore, every man has permanent aims and motives by which he guides his conduct, and he can always give an account of his particular actions; but if he were asked why he wills at all, or why in general he wills to exist, he would have no answer, and the question would indeed seem meaningless; and this would be just the expression of his consciousness that in itself is nothing but will, whose willing stands by itself and requires more particular determination by motives only in its acts at each point of time. In fact, freedom from all aim, from all limits, belongs to the nature of the will, which is endless striving.

It is imperative, in Schopenhauer's opinion, to strive to see through the deceptions, to untangle "the webs of the Maya." Anyone who succeeds in this will recognize himself in every other individual of the same species. It is only through this identification with others that one can achieve *Mitleid,* compassion, *agape, caritas, pietà.* "A person who has seen through the deception of the principles of individuation and has been able to free himself so that he can recognize his innermost self in all others will bring the endless suffering of others upon himself and will the affliction of the whole world."

Are we capable of such insight? Of course not. But can we strive toward that end? Yes, to a certain extent. What are the limits? When can we no longer endure? What exactly does "endure" mean? It means not to go under, to drown, to give up, but to continue until the night comes by itself, rather than rushing to meet it.

-Can we do this?
-Yes, to a certain extent.
-Is it worthwhile?
-I don't know. I don't understand what you mean by worthwhile.
-Should we try to do it?
-Stop saying "we." I can speak only for myself.
-The arrogance of the fatherless again?
-Yes, if you like.
-But what is your answer?
-Why do you call me "you"? Yes, if you insist on an answer, I will continue to try, as long as I can.
-Why?
-I don't know.
-Don't you realize that there are innumerable others, stronger, younger, better, wiser, more talented, ready to take over. They have already taken over, you are on your way out.
-Am I really on my way out? No, you are mistaken. Only a body with a certain name and registration number is on its way out, but not I.
-Isn't this body the prerequisite for even being able to say "I"?
-You keep calling me "you." Have we both fallen victim to the "veil of the Maya"?
-But what is your final word?
-That I know nothing. But I have the will.

Part Two: Suicides

2

Pista

O Mort, vieux capitane, il est temp! levons l'ancre!
Ce pays nous ennui, O Mort! Appareillons!

It's time now, Death, old sea captain! Cast off!
We weary of this land! Crowd all your sail!

Charles Baudelaire, "The Voyage"[1]

I have heard it said that the word "snow" is not used in the Same language, the language spoken in Lappland. A variety of different words can be used, depending on the type of snow and how one travels on it. Likewise, the Icelanders rarely use a single word for "lava," instead employing many different terms to describe various kinds of lava formations, their age, their shape, and the vegetation growing on them.

When I first began to learn Swedish, I was startled to realize that people talked about birch, pine, or spruce trees rather than simply "trees," as the city dwellers of Budapest did. My generation knew the names of hardly any of the different trees—a tree was merely a tree. My Swedish-born children have often criticized my meager horticultural vocabulary during our walks through the woods.

Hebrew, the only ancient language surviving in relatively unchanged form, has numerous expressions for sorrow, grief, worry, anxiety, and other troubled states of the soul, which seem to exceed the vocabulary of joy. Could this reflect the history of the Jewish people? Might it be equally characteristic of ancient languages that have become weakened and camouflaged as a result of the grammatical degeneration of most "modern languages"?

Another characteristic of Hebrew so strange to our ears is the nature of the verbs. In Latin and the Indo-European languages that have any grammar left to speak of, each verb is usually conjugated in only one way. But Hebrew verbs can be moved among seven different conjugation classes, and in doing so change their meaning, or at least their nuances. When the word "write" is moved to another conjugation group, it takes on the literal meaning "to induce someone to write," becoming the word "to dictate." Similarly, when the word "escape" is moved to another group, it comes to take on the meaning of helping someone or something escape, that is, to smuggle.

The verb *leabed* means to lose. Moving this word to another conjugation class changes the verb to *lehitabed*. This should literally mean "to lose oneself," but in both biblical and modern usage it has come to mean "to commit suicide."

Hebrew has several other equally meaningful expressions for suicide. "To do what causes loss of consciousness" is one such phrase. A third, painfully beautiful expression is "to lay hands on one's soul."

Pista and I were born less than two months apart.[2] I was the first grandchild in the family, Pista the second. Our fathers were brothers, the first and second of five children. I remained an only child, while Pista was joined by a little brother four years later. But we were close playmates throughout our childhood. In spite of the small age difference between us, everyone, including Pista and I, considered me the "older cousin."

I grew up in a somewhat more permissive environment than Pista. My father had died when I was a year and a half old, and my position as the only child of a widowed mother gave me certain privileges. There were few restrictions on me, for my mother had a basically liberal and supportive outlook on life, although one that reflected a rigidly defined perspective in some practical matters. Pista was also fairly unhampered, but his freedom was somewhat restricted by a series of German nannies whom his father, a well-known pediatrician, had hired and who had on occasion quite strict ideas about the way children should be disciplined. In one of my earliest memories, I can see a newly hired German girl taking five-year-old Pista and me out to play on Margareta Island. I can still see Pista refusing to eat a spinach dish from the container, the girl trying to force it into his mouth, Pista running around the bench screaming and crying, and the girl chasing in hot pursuit. I don't remember the outcome, but I do remember my joyous feeling of "I'm not part of this, I'm not in her power."

We spent our summers together in the home of our beloved grandmother, far from the city in Kaszony, the village of our fathers, on the Carpathian-Ukranian border. We played, rode our bicycles, played tennis, and generally did everything together. Our friendship had a somewhat reserved and intellectual foundation, and we never discussed our emotional lives, as if that part of us didn't exist. When I was twelve, I shared my newly discovered enthusiasm for music, and especially for opera, with Pista. He eventually became an equally devoted opera fan. We never went together—that was a private matter—but we always discussed our experiences afterward.

We shared the same room in grandmother's house, but we saw each other naked only once. That experience was associated with such an intense feeling of shame that I can still feel it to this day. The home of one of my uncles—originally the home of my father—was the only one in the village with "modern facilities," and we would use it once a week, at different times. Once, when we were about fourteen, the hot-water system had broken down, and we were told to use the bathhouse in the adjacent village. Unsuspectingly, we set out walking across the hills and through the vineyards. We stopped at a deserted farmhouse that had once belonged to our grandfather, and we talked about how our ancestors might have felt walking the same paths or riding in one of the horse carriages that were then still in use. We also discussed the important question of how far away in the valley the voice of Fiodor Chaliapin could be heard if he were standing on the mountaintop, singing. When we arrived at the bathhouse, we discovered that we would have to share the same bathroom, containing two old-fashioned bathtubs. We didn't have a chance to protest. We were given towels and soap, pushed into the room by a friendly woman, and the door was closed behind us. What an unbearable feeling of shame! We didn't talk about it, but I think we must have had the same feelings, for we both tried very hard to look away and not at each other. We quickly finished bathing and then tried to resume our conversation as usual, as if nothing had happened. (I was surprised when, fourteen years later, in the Swedish military, I discovered the natural behavior of boys together in a shower or sauna. Is this really the way it is? I then adapted quickly.)

We were in separate but more or less parallel classes in high school until we were sixteen. Our friendship remained close but hardly intimate. Our relationship began to deteriorate to some extent, however, when I realized that Pista's immediate family had often pointed to me as a role model for him to emulate. He didn't appreciate that. I started to play the piano, and so did Pista, although somewhat later. For a while he was more skillful than I, and he introduced me, among other things, to the music of Bela Bartók, a composer whose work was still very controversial. But I suspected that he considered me the "elder" and ahead of him, a feeling I disliked intensely. School grades were closely scrutinized in Pista's home, often with urgent requests for him to make more of an effort to improve. When I started to take private lessons in English—not exactly an acceptable language in the school system of fascist Hungary at the time—it was considered important for Pista to catch up with me, whether he wanted to or not. In fact, he did seem to want to, although his attitude toward me remained very positive. But there was a bit of a strain, a slight younger-brother complex. I had always longed for a younger brother, and I felt offended when I saw that my childhood friend and playmate had developed such a complex—even though I still did not have a younger brother. I kept to myself with my piano and my books, and sought out other friends.

Two years before graduation, when we were sixteen, our classes were fused, but by that time Pista and I had become almost strangers. Our relationship could be described as cool and polite. I had my own group of friends, with whom I discussed literature and poetry and went to the opera and concerts. Most of them were boys from school and from the same scout troop. Girls belonged to a different and segregated world, and the only contact possible with them was at dance school. But I refused to attend because I suspected, more or less justifiably, that I would have to endure bad music, superficial relationships, affected behavior, and empty conversation. Pista didn't attend either. His behavior was very

much like mine, but he didn't seem to have any friends whatsoever—he seemed completely isolated. He read a great deal, but
we talked less and less about our readings, our thoughts, and our
experiences.

Pista's alienation became more noticeable and was expressed
in more spectacular ways. He didn't seem to care any longer about
his classmates or his grades. The first "scandal" occurred when
we were assigned to write a paper on a subject of our choice,
dealing with something of great importance to us. All of my
friends despised our church-dominated, semi-fascist society and
its influence on the school system. Pista shared that feeling. Most
of us, however, thought that protests from us would be totally
meaningless, and we knew that we could not rely on any understanding from the corrupt and compliant majority of our teachers. We therefore chose to write about less current and controversial subjects. I wrote about "the role of the folk ballad in
nineteenth-century Hungarian poetry."

The moment the teacher entered the classroom with the corrected papers, we could see that he was terribly upset. He lectured
us sternly. One of the students had apparently written a paper for
which he really ought to be seen by the director and required to
face the school disciplinary committee, perhaps even be expelled
from school. Only the otherwise good behavior of the student
prevented the teacher from pursuing the matter further just then.
The paper was given a failing grade, something that had never
happened before.

It was Pista's paper. He accepted the failing grade without any
apparent emotion, but picked up the paper and tore it to pieces.
We managed to rescue only some fragments of it. It was covered
with angry red exclamation marks and emotional comments from
the teacher. From what was written on these small fragments and
from the little we managed to get out of Pista, we understood fairly
clearly that the paper was a devastating criticism of the entire
school system.

After this episode, Pista's grades plummeted and his reputation
deteriorated. He came to be considered a potentially disruptive
character. That assessment influenced all but two of his teachers.
One was Tibor Kardos, a humanitarian, a philosopher, a historian

of the Renaissance, and the only teacher left from the once-illustrious liberal tradition of our school. The other was the history teacher, a corrupt reactionary, a "lay priest" of the Catholic Church who, more than the others, should have been provoked by Pista's paper from an ideological point of view. But his children had been treated free of charge by Pista's father.

Grades were all-important as we began our last year at school. We had been forced, more or less reluctantly, to accept the view of our parents' generation that our school records were a matter of life and death. Without top grades, there was no chance for any further education. But neither we nor our parents could have imagined that we had been condemned to death by the world's most formidable military power, which had just conquered most of Europe and whose chances of final victory seemed highly probable. The history teacher, whose extra income from private lessons depended entirely on the Jewish students, or rather on their parents, discussed, for the sake of objectivity, his two alternative predictions for the future. One involved the presumed German victory, and the other a possible allied victory. He always added a *quod Deus avertat* —God forbid!—after the second possibility, and quickly crossed himself after uttering the three Latin words.

The months preceding graduation were characterized by maximal effort, particularly by the Jewish students who still had a chance to get good grades. After having spent the penultimate school year in a sort of daydream, absorbed in my music rather than showing an interest in school, I worked harder in my last year than perhaps at any other time in my life. Early in my teens I had gotten top grades, but during that previous year I dropped to a somewhat mediocre level. During the last year, my grades were again excellent. There wasn't time for anything except schoolwork, and I watched Pista, sitting only a few yards away from me in class, with a mixture of pleasant childhood memories and a certain degree of detachment. His own reserved behavior contributed to the sense of separation I felt. He didn't take part in the scramble for good grades, but his reserve was never expressed in any kind of aggressive behavior. Nevertheless, I sensed some slight condemnation of me, and that made me very sad. Our contacts became increasingly formal and infrequent.

I had hardly any social life at all, but although I never met any girls, I had already been initiated sexually two years earlier. Not at all reluctantly I had accompanied my closest classmates to "Madame Clarisse's" parlor, with a sense of curiosity yet with a certain feeling of detachment. The appearance, conduct, and refined speech of this venerable lady were in keeping with the best urbane traditions of both the Hungarian aristocracy and the cosmopolitan Jewish upper-middle class. She operated one of the "better" brothels in the central part of Budapest, which just happened to be located across the street from my piano teacher. On the door was a sign that read "Madame Clarisse," and her apartment did not really look any different from all the others, at least from the outside. Her many gentlemen customers were a fact of life. Young boys my age were encouraged to lie about how old they were—the legal age for admission was eighteen. Whenever the "adult" customers passed through the room in which we were sitting, after they had been let in somewhat surreptitiously, all the lights were turned off. "We wouldn't want you to meet your fathers here," Madame Clarisse said with a motherly wink. She was protective of us in other ways as well, and she let us in for a third of the usual price. "Let the old men pay—they can afford it," she used to say.

Pista never went with us on these outings, and he had never been to any other similar establishments, as far as I knew. But during our last school year, rumors began to circulate in class that he had been seen at a concert with a girl. Her name was Lia. She was the daughter of one of the richest Jewish merchants in town, and she was very beautiful. Some boys started to look at Pista with growing interest and a certain reluctant appreciation.

In the spring of 1943, during the most intensive period of preparation for our exams, the chamber choir in which I sang basso organized a private party. Naturally, because I didn't dance, I wasn't in the habit of going to parties. I was genuinely disgusted by the cacophony, smoke, liquor, bad music, and superficial conversation, all of which conspired to leave me with a bad headache. But on this occasion, the party had been organized by my beloved choir. Our director, Andras Korody, was only a few years older than I, and two decades later he became one of the most esteemed and internationally recognized conductors of the 1960s and 1970s. When he was no more than twenty or so, he already knew that he wanted to be a conductor, but because he was Jewish, he was barred from working with a choir or orchestra. He had therefore organized his own private chamber choir. We rehearsed once a week and performed in many of the rich Jewish homes in the hilly, beautiful sections of the city, singing everything from Orlando di Lasso to Zoltán Kodály, all a cappella. We were brought together by our music and by admiration for our conductor. This occasion was an anniversary of some kind, and our host rewarded our performance with a big party at his home on Svábhegy, the hill on which the Gestapo established their headquarters one year later. He encouraged us to bring friends.

I went to the party with a certain amount of pleasure and high expectations. But after a while, I found myself squeezed alone in a corner, bored and surrounded by the usual noise, dancing, and eating. It didn't seem to be any more engaging than any other party I had attended—perhaps it was my attitude that made them all seem the same.

Suddenly another of the bassos came up to me, accompanied by a beautiful dark girl with an open face. "This is Lia, she knows your cousin." I jumped up out of my chair, and Lia laughed. "What a quick move—just like a ski jumper," she said with gentle irony.

We began talking about Pista, and she mentioned that she used to go to concerts with him, but that she found him peculiar, severely introspective, and difficult to talk to.

We changed the subject. It turned out that both of us were fond of Thomas Mann. Because Lia had grown up partly in Vienna, she spoke German as readily as Hungarian. She was just then reading part four of Thomas Mann's work on Joseph and his sons, *Joseph der Ernährer* (*Joseph, the Provider*). The book had been published in Stockholm, but it was banned in Germany and its satellites. Nevertheless, it had reached Budapest through private channels. I was familiar with the first three books, and Lia told me about part four. We talked about opera, classical music, and mutual friends. To illustrate a point about a piece of music we had discussed, I sat down at the piano and played a few measures. Lia said that I had beautiful, nimble hands.

Toward the end of the evening, I was completely enchanted. On the way down in the cable tram, it was difficult for me to listen to the idle chatter of my colleagues in the choir, and I barely answered when they spoke to me. Previous conversations with other girls had been quite uninteresting, so different from my conversation with Lia that night.

We met again the next day, and I took her to the famous Russwurm café near the Buda castle. I had often heard of the café, but had never been there. Lia knew it quite well, and she wanted to have some of their chestnut puree. I realized that ordinarily the gentleman must pay the bill, but I had no idea how much the puree would cost. Did I have enough money? I knew that Lia was quite rich and that she never had any problem with money. I felt very embarrassed, and the conversation was quite forced until the bill arrived and I was relieved: I spent every penny I had, but at least I had enough!

We continued to see each other frequently, going to concerts and operas. Pista also went out with Lia, but his dates with her decreased as mine increased. I felt somewhat remorseful, but I couldn't resist her. We hardly ever touched, except for a light kiss once when we were on Margareta Island. Neither of us could imagine anything more intimate than that. Our behavior was typical of the pattern of youthful social interaction in central Europe. I went with Lia to her tennis lessons and admired her lovely figure and graceful flowing movements. Now and then, when it got to be too much, I visited Madame Clarisse's salon. But that didn't happen too often.

I also became a much more frequent visitor in Lia's home. Her parents, obese and overbearing people, took to me with great friendliness. They considered me a well-behaved young man with a good background and solid school achievements. Lia's father had rented the entire third floor of the Gresham Palace, an enormous architectural monument near the Chain Bridge on the Pest side of the river, near the Academy of Sciences. The building, now an office building, is as imposing a structure today in Budapest as it was then. The family also owned several other houses, all of them magnificently furnished for entertaining, card games, and empty conversation. To Lia and me both, that was a meaningless and wasteful sort of life. Lia didn't have particularly warm feelings for her father, one of the most important meat wholesalers in Austria and Hungary. He obviously favored her younger brother, a strikingly good-looking but spoiled and thoroughly unintellectual boy. But he was the great promise and was being groomed to take over the father's business. Lia was merely a girl, suitable only for decoration and for keeping company with socially acceptable families. But she was too intelligent, dynamic, and beautiful to tolerate that. She found escape in her interests in literature, poetry, and the company of many young men, including me. Despite the fact that I represented the opposite of everything her father stood for, her parents considered me socially acceptable. It was no coincidence that her first lover was one of Hungary's greatest poets, twenty years her senior and married to a musician. But that would happen two years later— a time still an ocean of German occupation, war, and deportations away. I would become the second, but that would be in the remote future, and it all seemed exceedingly unlikely at the time.

During the increasingly intense periods of study before graduation I saw Lia less frequently, but our meetings retained their intellectual tone. One day we were sitting in her summer house on Svábhegy mountain, not far from where we had first met. We were reading a chapter from Thomas Mann's fourth Joseph book, a part dealing with Tamar, the persistent young girl who sat at the feet of Jacob, listened to his tales, and decided to become the mother of all future generations of Jacob's tribe. She achieved that by dressing as a whore and seducing Judah, the heir, by the roadside. A wonderful biblical tale, written as only Thomas Mann could have. Lia was particularly taken in by Judah's claim that he was not really coveting lust, but that lust was seeking him.

Suddenly Lia looked out the window, and her face turned red.

"Here comes Pista," she said. "I told him that I don't want to see him anymore. Wait in the other room."

I waited. Their conversation was brief, and Lia came back in. Pista was already on his way out through the garden. I can still see his back—uncommunicative, ramrod straight, a body that moved without any apparent haste.

We continued to read about Tamar.

Graduation was approaching and all our thoughts centered on that. After a week of intensive written and oral examinations, we had a break of several days during which our grades were prepared. We were then called into the headmaster's office in alphabetical order, one after another, to receive our grades. My first name began with a G, Pista's with an I. He stood right behind me. I went in first, and I was pleased with my grades. I then waited for Pista, who stayed in the office an inordinately long time. Finally he came out, pale and quiet. "Well, how was it?" I asked. He showed me what he was holding in his hand—the graduation certificate torn to pieces. He had ripped it up himself, in front of the headmaster and the faculty. I could never find out why it took Pista so long to come out. He went to the wastepaper basket, threw away the certificate, and left.

That evening there was a big celebration party at a restaurant on Margareta Island. Strangely enough, Pista was also there, but he said nothing. There were some speeches, and we said goodbye to the teachers. We were feeling sentimental and already nostalgic for times we had shared in school, times that none of us appreciated while we were living them. Now we were on our way into "real life." In spite of the laws about Jews that had already been enacted, and the world war raging just outside our borders, none of us could even dream that two thirds of the Jewish boys would be killed in gas chambers and labor camps.

After the party, some of the boys got together to follow the school tradition by paying a visit to Madame Clarisse. I asked Pista if he wanted to come along. No, he said, and he went home.

After graduation, all of the Jewish students were drafted to work in the military labor camps, most of which were on the eastern front, deep in the Ukraine. They were forced to perform strenuous physical work under the most inhumane conditions, to support the hard-pressed German and Hungarian forces. We did not know that most members of these labor brigades were about to be annihilated, but we did know enough to try to avoid going. University students were granted deferrals. Hungary had been the very first country after the First World War to introduce a quota, "numerus clausus," for Jewish students. The quota for Jews was always far below the 10 percent representation of Jews in the country's population, but after the outbreak of the Second World

War—and particularly after the enactment of the so-called Jewish laws—it shrank to a trickle. Only the very best students, those with top grades and good connections, had the least chance for admission to the schools of law or economics. In some of the faculties, especially the medical schools, the number became "numerus nullus."

Both Pista and I had expressed an interest in studying medicine. I don't know why we harbored such a completely unattainable goal, because we were both much more interested in literature and music. Was it possible that our feelings for my uncle, Pista's father, had anything to do with it? I never met any of his patients, or any others with whom he dealt, no matter how fleetingly, who didn't love him—his calm, friendly, and confident manner; his kind hands; his smile and ability to avoid hurting anyone except when absolutely necessary. His own children loved him too, but not without a certain degree of regret and frustration. They could not talk with him as teenagers would like to, but usually cannot, talk with a father. Nonetheless, Pista wanted to study medicine, but it was just as impossible for him as it was for me. "Numerus nullus" prevailed, and only two Jewish boys in the whole country were admitted into the provincial medical schools, and even then only after extraordinary pressure from the highest political level.

Instead, we became "pseudo-medical students." Pista began by working as a volunteer in a clinical chemistry laboratory at the Jewish hospital. The purpose was to learn the basics for a possible later career in medicine, but he didn't really put his heart into it. Most of the time he sat at home, reading or writing I didn't know what. I was a "pseudo-law student," having been admitted to the law school at Pécs, a provincial university. I didn't have to attend the lectures, provided that I took my examinations at the appropriate time. I could therefore devote myself to my own personal interests, playing the piano and studying philosophy. I would have liked to have taken advantage of this academic freedom to attend the medical students' lectures, but Pécs was several hours away by train and my interest was obviously not intense enough to make the trip.

Lia and I met now and then. We went to concerts or for walks, keeping to the usual topics of conversation: literature, music, and mutual friends. We never mentioned Pista.

The war raged on close to our country, itself still idyllic and peaceful. Friends of mine who were a few years older were in the labor camps on the eastern front, and only a minority of them would survive. Several years earlier, the factories of death at Auschwitz, Treblinka, and Majdanek had already begun their daily annihilation of many thousands of Jews. Major new construction programs had recently begun at Auschwitz, including a fourth crematorium and additional railroad tracks to accommodate the last remaining contingents of European Jews, nearly a million of them from Hungary. But we knew nothing of this. We devoted ourselves to our own interests and didn't really notice anything special as we entered that fateful year of 1944, when 80 percent of the Jewish population of Hungary, including most of our relatives, would be murdered.

At the very beginning of the new year, the grandmother whom Pista and I both loved so much came to Budapest for a medical check-up. She brought with her our two-year-old cousin, the daughter of one of our uncles. Pista and I met again, and our somewhat chilled relationship was warmed for the last time by memories of our lost childhood years and the summers we spent together. As we waved goodbye to our grandmother, Pista said to me, "It's hard to believe that she is human. She is my idea of an angel."

I agreed. We had long since turned our backs on long words. We knew how hollow they were. We had disassociated ourselves from sentimental gestures. But in this case we knew that the expression was accurate, regardless of how and in what context it had been used by others. But we didn't know then that we had seen her and our little cousin for the last time.

A few days later, on January 9, as I was sitting at home reading, the door to the room opened. Pista came in, laughed a forced laugh, and handed me a sealed letter. He asked me to read it after he left and disappeared in a great rush.

I opened the letter. It was about ten pages long, handwritten in what seemed to be an agitated state. The letter opened with the comment that it could have been written only at night, when the constraints of the day had been erased.

I became apprehensive and skipped to the last page. The last words were, "When you have finished reading this letter, I will no longer be alive."

I threw down the letter and ran out as fast as I could. It was less than a mile to Pista's home. I rang the doorbell. His mother opened the door and saw how upset I was. Where's Pista? In the bathroom. I knocked on the door and began to shout. After a short while, Pista came out, laughing as if nothing had happened.

"How could you take that silly joke so seriously?"

I believed and disbelieved him at the same time. But I wanted to believe him, and I got very angry. How idiotic! Did he really think that he could gain people's sympathy in such a tawdry way? Don't we all need just as much sympathy?

On the way home I became really angry. Didn't Pista have anything better to do? When I got home, I threw away his letter without ever reading it thoroughly.

The next day I had a date with Lia. I told her what had happened, under the condition that she keep it confidential. Lia agreed that one shouldn't pay too much attention to such nonsense. We made plans to see a one-man performance by a famous actor a week later.

The performance took place on January 16 in the large hall of the Music Academy, and it was a tremendous disappointment. The much-admired actor, famous for his character roles, became a pitiful fool as he tried to read great poetry. There was not a single genuine feeling, not the slightest trace of insight into the hidden meanings in the poetry. It was turn-of-the-century romanticism at its worst. We went home extremely disappointed.

No sooner had I opened the door than I realized that something must have happened. The light was on, but my mother and stepfather were not at home. That had never happened before. Even more alarming was the fact that the apartment was a mess, as if its inhabitants, my pedantic mother and proper stepfather, had left in a great hurry. In fact, that is exactly what had happened. The beds were not made, and the doors of the closets were open. I wondered if they had been awakened. Why, by whom? My mother would never willingly leave her apartment in such a state.

As I was wondering whom I should call, the door opened. My mother and stepfather came in, deathly pale, trembling, beside themselves with desperation. I had never seen them like that.

What happened? Pista is dead.

He had been sitting at his desk as usual during the afternoon, staring at the skull he had gotten some time before. It was a real skull, not an imitation; he had said that he wanted to study the anatomy of the skull to prepare for the medical studies he hoped were to come. When his father looked into the room to tell Pista that dinner was ready, he found his son with his head on the desk. Only when he came closer did he see that Pista was lying with his head in a pool of blood. Next to him was a small air pistol, the kind used to shoot at birds, half seriously, half for fun. With luck, birds shot with this kind of gun could survive. But Pista was dead.

An inquiry later revealed that Pista had bought the pistol at the flea market. It was the kind of gun for which a license was not required. He studied the skull carefully to find where the bone was the thinnest, and shot himself exactly there. The bullet happened to hit a major blood vessel.

A sense of darkness, nausea, and unreality, combined with a reluctance to believe what I had heard, are the feelings that come to mind when I try to reconstruct my immediate reaction. But above all, I remember a desperate feeling of wanting to go back in time, to start all over again from the beginning, to undo it all.

I grabbed the telephone. Lia answered. I told her what I had just heard. After a very brief pause came her nonchalant voice: "Will you release me now from your ban?" At first I didn't understand what she meant, but I soon realized that she was referring to the promise of secrecy I had imposed on her about Pista's unexpected visit the previous week. I was furious—is that all you can say? Can't you think of anything else? You are really heartless—I don't want to see you ever again.

I hung up. We didn't meet again until two years later, after the war, the deportations, and the mass murders had placed additional layers of tragedy onto Pista's death.

But at the time I had no idea of all that was to come. For days and weeks I walked around as if in a trance with Pista's brother, four years younger.

We searched through Pista's drawers, reading papers he had left behind. I tried to comprehend the incomprehensible, all the time also trying to answer questions from a world that understood even less than I did. But most difficult of all was my inner dialogue:

Could I have prevented it, if only I had taken the first warning more seriously? Every one of those "discussions" ended with an unequivocal "yes."

Pista's drawers were filled with papers—poems and more poems, a whole volume. They had all been written during the previous three years, including our last two years at school. And I had no idea. What poetry! After a faltering start, he had suddenly found his full voice, achieving a level of literary expression that needed only to take the next few steps on the road to mastery. But with literary maturation one could discern a growing alienation, a pessimism that included all the available expressions in the language for hopelessness, for the total lack of meaning, progressing steadily toward increasing darkness, while still full of nostalgia for a life already long passed, a life never to return. The idyll of childhood, perhaps? The optimism of early adolescence? His last poems spoke of death as the only possible deliverance. Many years later, I read the poetry of another victim of suicide, Paul Celan:

Schwarze Milch der Frühe wir trinken sie abends
wir trinken sie mittags und morgens wir trinken sie nachts
wir trinken und trinken
wir schaufeln ein Grab in den Lüften da liegt man nicht eng

Black milk of daybreak we drink it at sundown
we drink it at noon in the morning we drink it at night
we drink and we drink it
we dig a grave in the breezes there one lies unconfined

These lines from his *Todesfuge* ("Death Fugue") brought Pista's poems to mind—they are so similar in tone and feeling. But Celan was writing about Auschwitz ("death is a master from Germany, his eyes are blue") from which he could never release himself, while Pista was writing from the subconscious idyllic level of our happy-unhappy childhood. What would he have done if he had lived two more months, until the German invasion? Would he have recovered his will to live, only to defy death, the master from Germany with the blue eyes? Or would he have succumbed anyway?

Pista's brother and I went to visit the only teacher we respected, Tibor Kardos. He read some of the poems and bowed his head into his hands. He was especially impressed with one of the last poems, entitled "Maimed Column," and was convinced that Pista would have become a great poet. We ought to talk with a publisher, he suggested. He felt that the collection of poems was ready for publication, and that they should be published under that same title. We had just made our first tentative contacts with a publisher when the German invasion began on March 19, sweeping away everything.

But Pista's memory lingers deeply buried in my consciousness, surfacing now and then.Would I have been able to prevent his death? The answer is always the same—yes, you could have done that, you were the only one who might have prevented it, if only you had taken him seriously, if only you could have controlled the irritation you felt with him. But what was it that really annoyed me? The incessant attempts by those around us to compare us, to portray me as a role model for him, must have aroused his sense of resentment and anger, alienating him from me and therefore, me from him. When I, that same role model, sat after Pista's death reading some of those wonderful poems—written during the night with exaggerated large letters—finally able to understand something of the volcano concealed underneath that private facade, I felt more ashamed than I had ever thought possible. I wanted only to sink into the crater of that erupting volcano and disappear. We had been like brothers for many years, two different, seemingly individual manifestations of the common commodity of our species. The courses of our lives had run closely together. How was it possible that in my self-centered journey I had strayed so far from him, unaware of the fate of the brother who had been so close to me?

At the funeral Pista's brother and I walked together. We talked about the inevitability of death, an idea we accepted but at the same time wanted to ignore. I suddenly felt that there were only three ways to survive this dilemma: to believe in spiritualism or other similar nonsense, to rationalize away the whole matter and claim that I had no more responsibility than anyone else, or to store it away as what it really was, an incurable wound deep in my consciousness.

3

Attila József

Lídi nénémnek öccse itt,
Batu Kán pesti rokona,
Kenyéren élte éveit
s nem volt azúrkék paplana;
Kinek verséért a halál
Öles kondérban főz babot—
hejh burzsoá! hejh proletár!
én, József Attila, itt vagyok!

Kid brother of my Aunt Lidi,
Khan Batu's kinsfolk in Budapest,
Bread was his food over the years,
never owned an eiderdown, blue like the sea;
For whose poems
cooks beansoup in a large cauldron—
hi bourgeois! hi proletarian!
I, Attila József I'm right here![1]

In Hungarian, a person's family name is written first, before the given name. In the case of Attila József, either József or Attila can be used as a first name. The foreign style of writing a name, given name first, appears strange to a Hungarian-speaking person, especially when one is referring to a well-known figure. In Hungarian, he is called József Attila, but in English or most other languages we would call him Attila József, or Attila for short.

It is difficult to travel through any town or city in contemporary Hungary without finding a street, a square, or a park named after József Attila. Statues of him stand in many places, and several museums are named for him. The university in Szeged that once expelled him is now called József Attila University.

Arthur Koestler, whose mother tongue was Hungarian, considered Attila the greatest poet of the century. In his autobiography, *Invisible Writing,* Koestler says:

The unique quality of the poems of his later years lies in their miraculous union of intellect and melody. In this respect I can think of no contemporary poet to whom he could be compared. His most complex and cerebral Marxist and Freudian poems read like folk-songs, and sometimes like nursery rhymes; "ideology" is here completely distilled to music which, whether *adagio* or *furioso,* is always eminently *cantabile.* His rhythm almost automatically translates itself into song; his rhymes are virgin matings of rolling four- and five-syllable words . . . all of which turns translating into a nightmare of frustration.[2]

In the late fall of 1937, after having spent several months in a private hospital under psychiatric care, the thirty-two-year-old Attila was visiting his two sisters near Lake Balaton. One day he took a walk to the railway station. He had always been fascinated by trains and often used them in his poetry. As a freight train began to slowly pull out of the station, Attila threw himself between the cars. The news of his death and the description of his badly mangled body was brought to the sisters by the giggling village idiot.

Who was Attila? What does his poetry say to past and present generations of Hungarians? How can his work, in just a few seconds, so transform my own consciousness—I, a naturalized Swede for more than forty years?

He belonged to all of us and none of us. During his short life he suffered all the infernal torments that such a tortured psyche can endure, but nevertheless he was able to laugh at his pain. One of his collections, written when he was twenty-four, begins with "Hip, hop!" and continues:

Like an anecdote
on the skirts of well-stacked peasant girls
you come and go under the sky
the semi flat-footed Attila
of the beats;
and on your ragged and fading lowers
where you wear the Order of the Golden Fleece
they stare wide of mouth—the goats, the bears,
and girls! little old women! sunflowers!

Almost everyone who reads Attila's poetry in the original Hungarian will come to a complete stop just there, and simply stare. One needn't be a virgin or a sunflower to do so, but one must know Hungarian. Who was he, why did he write as he did—why did he quit life so early, why did he die by his own hand?

Before we begin searching for answers to these questions, we might try to hear his own voice behind the almost impenetrable language barrier. I have chosen to start with a poem that immediately grabs me, no matter how often I have read it or what my mood is. No translation can do more than hint at its meaning or convey its exhilarating poetic power and rhythmic precision. It was written in 1932, when the poet was twenty-seven years old.

The Seventh

If you set out in this world,
better be born seven times.
Once, in a house on fire,
once, in a freezing flood,
once, in a wild madhouse,
once, in a field of ripe wheat,
once, in an empty cloister,
and once among pigs in a sty.
Six babes crying, not enough:
you yourself must be the seventh.

When you must fight to survive,
let your enemy see seven
One, away from work on Sunday,
one, starting his work on Monday,
one, who teaches without payment,
one, who learned to swim by drowning,
one, who is the seed of a forest,
and one, whom wild forefathers protect,
but all their tricks are not enough:
you yourself must be the seventh.

If you want to find a woman,
let seven men go for her,
One, who gives his heart for words,
one, who takes care of himself,
one, who claims to be a dreamer,
one, who through her skirt can feel her,
one, who knows the hooks and snaps,
one, who steps upon her scarf:
let them buzz like flies around her.
You yourself must be the seventh.

If you write and can afford it,
let seven men write your poem.
One, who builds a marble village,
one, who was born in his sleep,
one, who charts the sky and knows it,
one, whom words call by his name,
one, who perfected his soul,
one, who dissects living rats.
Two are brave and four are wise;
you yourself must be the seventh.

And if all went as was written,
you will die for seven men.
One, who is rocked and suckled,
One, who grabs a hard young breast,
one, who throws down empty dishes,
one, who helps the poor to win,
one, who works till he goes to pieces,
one, who just stares at the moon.
The world will be your tombstone:
you yourself must be the seventh.[3]

Five times six, thirty altogether. Attila has played all thirty roles in his poem, and he tried to live accordingly. But who were the remaining five—where do we find the seventh? Why did he choose that very word, "one whom words call by its first name, one who throws down empty dishes?"

In the spring of 1937, half a year before his horrible suicide, Attila prepared and submitted a curriculum vitae as part of an application for a job as an office clerk. He was born in Budapest in 1905, to a Greek Orthodox family. At the time there were very few Greek Orthodox living in Hungary. Most people were Catholic, Protestant, or Jewish. He wrote that his father, Aron Jósef, emigrated to America when Attila was only three years old. But in fact, Attila had been deceived on that point. Subsequent studies showed that the Rumanian Aron Jusef abandoned his wife and three children—two girls, Jolán and Eta, and the youngest, the son Attila—and settled down with another woman in Rumania. By spreading false rumors, he wanted to fool his wife into thinking that he had left for the United States. With the help of a child-protection agency, Attila was placed in a temporary foster home in the countryside. He continued: "I lived there until I was seven years old. I started to work at a very early age, like most of the other poor children who lived in the rural areas, herding swine." His foster parents refused to call him Attila because they had consulted with their neighbors and concluded that there was no such name. Instead, they gave him the very common name Pista. Attila was badly shaken by this, because he felt that they were casting doubt on his very existence.

When Attila was seven his mother, Borbála Pöcze, took the three children with her to Budapest. She was the sole provider for her family, working as a laundress and charwoman. Attila was enrolled into the second grade of elementary school. It was there that he first read about the king of the Huns, and he was elated by the discovery that the name Attila actually existed. According to him, it was this childhood experience that kindled his interest in literature and made him a thinker, willing to listen to the views of others but accepting them only after scrutinizing them himself.

Attila was nine when the First World War erupted. His family's existence grew increasingly miserable. The young boy was often forced to stand in line at the food store from nine in the evening until eight-thirty the following morning, only to hear, when his turn finally came, that all the food had been sold. He tried by all conceivable means to be of help. He sold drinking water at the movie theater, The Globe, stole firewood and coal from the nearby freight-train station, made colored paper pinwheels and sold them to the wealthier children, carried packages and baskets at the market, sold newspapers, and traded stamps. But in 1918 the family's plight grew even worse. His mother was hospitalized with uterine cancer and was allowed home for only brief periods of time. Shortly after the end of the war, during the temporary Rumanian occupation, Attila worked as a waiter in one of the large cafés. At that time he enrolled in a four-year district high school, one that was intended for students who wanted more than the four-year elementary school but who were not sufficiently motivated, competent, or wealthy to attend the eight-year program at the (junior-college level) *gymnasium.*

In his curriculum vitae, the fourteen-year-old Attila devoted only two sentences to two enormous changes that took place in his life in 1919; his mother died, and his brother-in-law, Dr. Ödön Makai, was named his guardian. Several important studies have been carried out on this period of Attila's life, most notably the extensive writings by the literary scholar Miklos Szabolcsi (*Fiatal életek indulója*, Budapest, 1963: *Érik a fény*, Budapest, 1979). The short-lived communist rule was followed by Admiral Horthy's semi-fascist counterrevolutionary regime. For Attila it was a time of deepening despair—his mother's incurable illness, the misery of his existence in the slums, the unending lines for a piece of bread or a glass of milk for his mother.

The divorce of his older sister Jolán and her subsequent marriage to the well-off Jewish lawyer Makai were decisive events for Attila, but in a different sort of way. Makai was the "black sheep" of a successful middle-class family. He fostered Jolán's education with the kind of attention reminiscent of Professor Higgins's devotion to Eliza Doolittle in Shaw's play "Pygmalion." The intelligent proletarian girl was transformed within a remarkably short time into a well-dressed middle-class lady of refined speech and conduct. But she was not accepted by her husband's family. Makai tried to conceal her humble origins from their circle of friends and acquaintances, and his rather ambivalent attitude toward the younger sister Eta and Attila must be viewed from this perspective. They were permitted to live with their brother-in-law for a period, but whenever visitors came to the house, Eta and Attila were introduced as temporary servants. Makai was generous with Attila's school expenses, but otherwise wanted to have as little as possible to do with him.

Attila soon escaped back into the slums. During summer vacations and even during part of the school year, he worked on river tugboats. From Szabolcsi's detailed biography we learn that Attila performed the most menial kinds of work. He scrubbed the decks of the tugs, and although it was a monotonous and badly paid job, it didn't interfere with preparations for final examinations at the secondary school he had been able to attend on a somewhat irregular basis.

After completing his final year in school, he was sent by his guardian to a Catholic seminary as a novice, where he was not well received. He was, after all, officially Greek Orthodox, and that weighed heavily against him. He could endure only two weeks there. He was admitted to a boarding school in Makó in the Hungarian lowlands, not far from the university town of Szeged.

Makó was then the center of the onion-growing region of Hungary and was populated mostly by farmers, many of them quite wealthy. Attila writes only briefly about this period of his life, mentioning only that he was granted cost-free tuition at school and that he took on tutoring to pay for his room and board. But his biographers have much more to tell. He was an outsider, a strange bird among the sons of the prosperous landowners and civil servants. He went around in ill-fitting and patched old clothes donated to him by his brother-in-law and sister. Oddly enough, his clothing was shabby but, at the same time, pretentious. He felt lonely and abandoned, preferring to remain in town even during holidays and school vacations. His behavior and fervent interest in his studies aroused deep suspicion and rumors that he might be illegitimate, a profound stigma in that highly conservative farming society.

Attila read voraciously and as early as his teens was writing poetry. By the time he was fifteen, he had earned the nicknames "Mister" and "The Poet" and was being noticed by his teachers as well as by the groups organized by the more ambitious students. Of his time in Makó, he wrote:

I finished high school with excellent grades in all subjects, despite puberty problems and several attempts at suicide. That was not surprising, given the fact that I didn't have any good friends to guide me. When I was seventeen, my first poems were published in *Nyugat*.[4] I was looked upon as a child prodigy, but in reality I was merely an orphan.

Attila received the highest grades whether or not he paid attention to his teachers, but he decided to leave before finishing high school. He felt not only forsaken, but also idle. He began working as a day laborer in the cornfields and continued tutoring the unintelligent children of local well-to-do families. Two teachers who had become personally attached to Attila persuaded him to return to school, and after an additional year of private study he graduated a year ahead of his former classmates. But even before that he had been brought into court on charges of blasphemy, based on one of his poems. He was initially found guilty by a lower court, but an appeals court reversed the decision and acquitted him.

After graduation Attila was employed as a bank clerk, but he was subjected to constant harassment by his more senior colleagues.

They foisted their own work on him and ridiculed his poetry. "When I was your age, I wrote poetry too," they remarked. It was then that he decided to make a serious attempt to become a writer and tried to find a solid middle-class job that he could combine with his literary work and that would allow him to maintain contact with the world of letters. But he also wanted to continue his studies, and so he enrolled in the faculty of humanities at the University of Szeged, majoring in Hungarian and French litera-ture. He took fifty-two hours of classes per week, and completed more than half of his coursework with distinction. He lived on the edge of starvation, with only the meager royalties from his poetry as income. One of his professors urged him to begin some independent research work.

But his university studies came to a sudden and unexpected halt. Professor Horger, one of Attila's examiners in Hungarian philology, summoned him and announced, in the presence of two witnesses, that as long as it was in his power, he would see to it that Attila would never be allowed to sit for the qualifying examination for a high school teaching position. Holding up that day's newspaper, Horger declared, "A person who writes this kind of poetry is not to be trusted with the education of the new generation."

This is the poem that was condemned by Horger:

Innocent Song

I have no God, I have no king,
my mother never wore a ring,
I have no crib or funeral cover,
I give no kiss, I take no lover.

For three days I have chewed my thumb,
for want of either crust or crumb.
Though I am twenty, strong and hale—
my twenty years are up for sale.

Should there be none who wish to buy,
The devil's free to have a try;
then shall I use my common sense
and rob and kill in innocence.

Till, on a rope, they hang me high,
and in the blessed earth I lie—
and lush and poisoned grasses start
rank from my pure and simple heart.[5]

Koestler's translation is fairly good, but it still misses the remarkable musical quality of Attila's language, which Koestler caught so well in his opening quotation. I would like to give the non-Hungarian reader at least some feeling for this quality. Please try to read aloud the first and last four lines in the original Hungarian. The Hungarian language is generally pronounced phonetically, but some of the letters stand for sounds different from those in English. The letter "s" is pronounced "sh," sz is pronounced "s," "gy" is pronounced like a "d," just as you sometimes hear it in the middle of the word "Magyar" (there is no corresponding sound in the English language), and "cs" is pronounced "ch" as in the word "chalk." The letter "a" is pronounced as the "o" in "one," whereas "á " is pronounced as the "a" in "cart." The letter "ö" is similar to the sound of the letter "i" in "bird." In all words, the first syllable is accented.

Nincsen apám, se anyám
se istenem, se hazám
se bölcsöm, se szemfedöm
se csókom, se szeretöm

Elfognak és felkötnek
áldott földdel elfödnek
s halált hozó fü
gyönyörüszép szivemen

The eminent literary scholar Lajos Hatvany has called this poem a "documentation of the post-war generation, a poem that will survive for a very long time." And it has done just that. A well-known Hungarian author who published under the pseudonym "Ignotus" has written in *Nyugat* that he has "murmured, whispered, sung, caressed and cradled this miraculously beautiful poem" that time and again came into his mind. He chose it as the motto for his own book, *Ars poetica*, considering it an outstanding example of the new era in poetry.

After his encounter with Horger, Attila saw no point in continuing with his teacher's training. Horger held a prominent position in Hungary's feudal educational system, and his attitudes reflected the ideological climate of the time, which left no room for student protests. Twelve years later, only a few months before he committed suicide, Attila returned to this episode in a poem that he wrote for his thirty-second birthday:

On My Birthday
I am thirty-two and wise.
Poem, be a big surprise
   pretty
   ditty.

Gift that shall my spirit rouse
in the lonely coffeehouse
   who? me
   who? me.

Thirty-second, whizzing by.
Ten a week? I only try,
   shaft me,
   Hungary!

Could have been an educator
but became a pencil nibbler
   sure
   poor.

One fine day they ousted me
from the university
   fool
   school.

They expelled me forth and hence
for my "Song of Innocence"
   fending
   sending.

He defended Hungary,
rules of the Academy
   name
   shame.

"Long as I am teaching here
stay clear of this hemisphere"
   gloating
   bloating.

If Professor Horger's glad
poet's grammar turns out bad
   little
   spittle.

Mine's a school for all the people,
not the high school pap and nipple,
   each in,
   teach in![6]

After his expulsion from the Szeged university, Attila went to Vienna, where he enrolled at the university and supported himself by selling newspapers at the Rathauskeller restaurant and being a janitor at the Collegium Hungaricum. By chance, the director, Antal Lábán, learned that the new janitor was the poet whose work he knew so well. He invited Attila for dinner at the Collegium and arranged employment for him as a private tutor. After spending the night at a shelter for the homeless poor, without even a sheet covering his bed, Attila was invited to spend the summer in the castle of the literature-loving Baron Bertalan Hatvany in the Hungarian countryside. With some funds from his brother-in-law, Attila was able to continue his studies at the Sorbonne in Paris. Soon thereafter he wrote the short poem entitled "Picture Postcard from Paris":

A patron never rises in the morning
In Paris Jeanettes are Berthas and
a man can buy cooked spinach
or burning candles at the barbershop.

Sixty naked women sing to heaven
all the way down to St. Michel
and Notre Dame: it's cold inside,
and for five francs you can see me from above.

The Eiffel tower tilts toward the night
and nestles under quilted fog,
a policeman will kiss you if you're a girl
and there are no toilet seats in the restrooms.[7]

After his stay in Paris, Attila spent two semesters studying at the University of Budapest, but he didn't try to work toward his teacher's diploma. He considered it useless, because he believed that it would be impossible to get a job in the face of Horger's threat. The last part of Attila's career and his curriculum vitae are quite brief, indicating a rather chaotic existence. He wrote that he tried his hand at several temporary jobs, and even listed a number of references. But because of "unexpected blows," he was hospitalized several times. "I wasn't able to endure these setbacks, no matter how life had toughened me. Since then, my only income came from my writings." At the end of his curriculum vitae, he lists all his qualities: reads and writes Hungarian, French,

German; experienced in Hungarian and German business correspondence; perfect typist; knowledgeable in shorthand and in the
techniques of printing. He continues, "I consider myself honest;
I think I learn quickly and can work hard."

The Poet and His Work

Countless books and articles have been published in Hungary
during the past half century dealing with some aspect of the
phenomenon of Attila József. One particularly important piece
of work was published in 1982 by two psychologists and a literary
expert, all thirty-two years old—Attila's age at the time of his
death. The precise title of this book was *It Was in the Midst of You
That I Became Mad,*[8] a quotation from one of his last poems. The
book deals partly with Attila's last years, to which we will return
later in the section on his illness and death, and partly with his
poetry and its multifaceted impact on Hungarian literature.
During Attila's lifetime, his writing was appreciated by only a
relatively small number of people, but the group expanded
markedly after his death. It wasn't until the 1970s that he finally
became one of the most important figures in the rich fabric of
Hungarian poetry. His work is now regarded as paradigmatic of
his time.

It seems as if Attila's poetry had been lying in wait for the
historically appropriate moment, almost half a century after he
started his career as a poet, when it was finally able to break
through and reach far beyond the small circle of literati. His work
has been experienced by many Hungarians as documentation of
their own past and their roles in life. The feeling that Attila's
poetry is "about all of us" has spread like ripples on the surface
of a pond. His poetry forces readers to constantly question their
own situations, to examine who they are and who they would have
or should have become. It is easy to identify with the poet. Readers
try to build bridges between the work and the fate of the poet,
between the poetry and their own individual positions in life.

If one were to search for a unifying thread in this radiant life's
work, one would find two central motifs: the question "Who am
I?" and the struggle for growth and self-realization. The suffering
produced by a journey through an individual hell is looked upon

as an obvious and inevitable prerequisite for maturity and personal growth. Attila was forced to suffer much more than most,
even during his early childhood, and his mental suffering continued throughout his life. For a collection of poems that he published in 1934 under the title *The Bear Dance,* Attila chose a motto
taken from a folk song: "He who wants to learn how to play the
bagpipe must first enter into Hell; there and only there can he
learn how the pipe is to be played."

Freedom and responsibility, maturity, and earnestness are some
of the key words of this starving proletarian writer, one whose
yearning for the love of his mother and of other women haunted
him all his life. One year before his death he wrote:

A Breath of Air

Who can forbid my telling what hurt me
    on the way home?
Soft darkness was just settling on the grass,
    a velvet drizzle,
and under my feet the brittle leaves
tossed sleeplessly and moaned
    like beaten children.

Stealthy shrubs were squatting in a circle
    on the city's outskirts.
The autumn wind cautiously stumbled among them.
    The cool moist soil
looked with suspicion at streetlamps;
a wild duck woke clucking in a pond
    as I walked by.

I was thinking, anyone could attack me
    in that lonely place.
Suddenly, a man appeared,
    but walked on.
I watched him go. He could have robbed me,
    since I wasn't in the mood for self-defence.
I felt crippled.

They can tap all my telephone calls
    (when, why, to whom).
They have a file on my dreams and plans
    and on those who read them.
And who knows when they'll find
sufficient reason to dig up the files
    that violate my rights.

In this country, fragile villages,
    —where my mother was born—
have fallen from the tree of living rights
    like these leaves
and when a full-grown misery treads on them
a small noise reports their misfortune
    as they're crushed alive.

There is not the order I dreamed of. My soul
    is not at home here
in a world where the insidious
    vegetate easier,
among people who dread to choose
and tell lies with averted eyes
    and feast when someone dies.

This is not how I imagined order.
    Even though
I was beaten as a small child, mostly
    for no reason,
I would have jumped at a single kind word.
I knew my mother and my kin were far,
    these people were strangers.

Now I have grown up. There is more foreign
    matter in my teeth,
more death in my heart. But I still have rights
    until I fall apart
into dust and soul, and now that I've grown up
my skin is not so precious that I should put up
    with the loss of my freedom.

My leader is in my heart. We are
    men, not beasts,
we have minds. While our hearts ripen desires,
    they cannot be kept in files.
Come, freedom! Give birth to a new order,
teach me with good words and let me play,
    your beautiful serene son.[9]

Yes, that is exactly what he hoped to be—the beautiful and
serene son of freedom—he, the most playful of all poets, who
could amaze his readers by amalgamating concepts, visions, ideas,
and facts from seemingly unrelated areas and condensing them
into a few well-crafted sentences. These may appear inordinately
compressed at first sight, but they have a strange potential to burst
open suddenly after some reflection, like a flower, leaving the
reader stunned, moved, and unable to decide what to admire

more, the beauty of the poet's language or the logical clarity of his thought. His sentences could be surrealistic or plain like the language of a child; he could create huge magical figures from poor peasants or factory workers living in filthy slums. But above all, he could transfigure the image that he uses most often in his writing, the worn-out mother, dying of cancer:

Mother

She held her mug with both hands
one Sunday, and with a quiet smile
she sat a little while
in the growing dusk.

She brought home in a tiny skillet
the food they gave her where she worked.
Going to bed I kept thinking—
the rich always fill their bellies.

My mother was a small woman.
She died early, as washerwomen do:
their legs tremble from carrying,
their heads ache from ironing.

For mountains they have the dirty laundry.
Their cloudscapes are made of steam.
And if they want a change of climate,
they can climb the attic stairs.

I see her pausing with the iron.
Her frail body, grown thinner and thinner,
was broken by capital.
Think about this, proletarians.

She was stooped from all that laundry.
I didn't realize she was a young woman.
In her dreams she wore a clean apron
and then even the mailman said hello.[10]

In his writings, correspondence, and conversations, Attila repeatedly emphasized that "striving for earnestness" is the most important task for a young poet. He recognized, however, that it could not be achieved by tranquil contemplation, but must come through constant questioning, through an incessant struggle with oneself and with society. Attila's struggle stemmed from his background and social circumstances. Hungary under Admiral Horthy was a feudal, semi-fascist state, forged by centuries of conflict among the variety of social classes, ethnic groups, and

religions. Those of the privileged class unscrupulously domi-
nated the backward and impoverished masses. No one was concerned about Ferencváros (Franzstadt), the proletarian district
where Attila was born and grew up, where he starved and froze,
labored and stole before his poetry came to be recognized and
honored by the established masters of the language. Attila brought
the outskirts of the city into the limelight; his literary metaphors
were suddenly on everyone's lips.

Night on the Outskirts

Slowly the light's net is lifted
Out of the yard, and our kitchen
Fills with darkness
Like the hollows deep in a pool.

Silence—
The scrubbing brush creeps to life,
Above it, a patch of wall
Hesitates, hangs, not sure
Whether to stay or fall.

A night that wears oily rags
Heaves a sigh,
Halts in the sky;
Then settles on the outskirts,
Waddles over the square
And lights a bit of moon to see by.

Like ruins the factories loom.
But inside them a denser gloom
Even now is being produced. It sets,
A foundation for silence.

Through the windows of textile mills
Fly moonbeams in sheaves—
Moon thread till morning weaves
On motionless looms a fabric
Of girl worker's dreams.

Farther on, like a cloistered graveyard,
The foundry, bolt makers, cement works—
Echoing family crypts.
Too well these workshops keep
The secret of resurrection.

A cat's claws on the fence;
And the simple night watchman sees
A ghost, a flashing signal.
Cooly gleam
The beetle-backed dynamos.

A train whistle blows.

Dampness seeps into
The shadows, the boughs
Of a fallen tree.
The dust on the road grows heavy.

In the street a policeman,
A muttering workman, pass.
Now and then a comrade
Flits past with leaflets—
Keen as a dog on the track ahead
Listening, cat-like, for noises behind him;
avoiding the lamps.

The tavern door belches out
A tainted light, its windows
Vomit, leaving puddles.
Inside, a half-stifled lamp
Slowly swings,
A solitary labourer keeps awake.
While the innkeeper snores and wheezes,
He bares his teeth at the wall,
His grief climbs the stairs. He weeps,
Cries out for the revolution.

Cold metal, the water clinks.
A stray mongrel, the wind
Wanders. Its great tongue hangs
To touch the water, and laps it.
Straw mattresses are the rafts
That drift on night's currents.

The warehouse's hulk is aground.
In the foundry's iron dinghy
The smelter dreams red babies
Into the metal molds.

All is damp, and heavy.
Mildew draws a map
Of misery's regions.
And there, on the dry meadows,
Rags and paper litter
The ragged, papery grass.
How they would whirl and fly!
They stir, but inertia holds them.

Night, your sluggish breeze
Is a flapping of soiled sheets.
Like frayed muslin to cord
You cling to the old sky,

As wretchedness clings to life.
Night of the poor, be my coal,
Smolder here on my heart,
Melt the iron in me, to make
An anvil that never will split
A hammer that clangs and glints,
A smooth blade for victory, night!

Grave this night is, and heavy.
I too shall sleep now, my brothers.
May our souls not be smothered by want.
Nor our bodies be bitten by vermin.[11]

Attila became an overt revolutionary and the only proletarian
Hungarian writer able to describe the desperate plight of the
poor in a society that preferred to ignore the problem. But his
form of socialism was odd and idiosyncratic, intolerant of any sort
of party discipline. He was only temporarily accepted by the
harshly disciplinary apparatus of the illegal Communist Party
organization, of which he was a member until he was expelled.
He must have felt as much out of place there as a soaring seagull
at a military air maneuver.

The confrontation between real life and an artificial, mindless,
and hostile society is a constantly recurring theme in Attila's work.
In the beginning of one of his most famous revolutionary poems,
"On the City Limits Where I Live," composed in 1933, he writes:

the soot settles
softwinglike, batlike
and ossified like guano
hard and slow.

Thus weighs this age on our chests.
Like graymops of rain
swabbing
the jagged roofs of tin,
a sorrow in vain
poultices the crust of our pain.[12]

The poet alone is a recorder of history. Only he can look
consciously into the future, only he can "edit" the subjective
harmony and convey it with his "rattling lips" to "you out there
in the objective sphere." This is the only way to realize "our
wonderful ability to create order, so that our thoughts can con-

ceive our limited infinity, the productive forces outside and the instincts inside."

Those who live in the peaceful and democratic societies of the 1990s may have some trouble understanding how revolutionary these ideas were in the 1920s and 1930s. The counterrevolution-ary government of Horthy that crushed Béla Kun's aborted communist regime following the collapse of the Hungarian monarchy was certainly more benign and "respectable" than the fascist dictatorships in Italy and Germany. Nevertheless, the unholy alliance of Hungarian landowners, the aristocracy, and the military led to the domination of a corrupt and unscrupulous privileged class. The signing of the ethnographically ruthless Trianon Peace Treaty led to the emergence of extreme and often anti-Semitic nationalist movements, collectively called "the awak-ening Hungarians," many of which arose in the universities. They preached a kind of "moral rearmament" and were often sup-ported by the Catholic Church. They despised the liberal cultural movements from the West and were hostile toward the cosmopoli-tan culture of the capital. They tried to create a variety of patriotic myths, all quite confused. It was against the background of such a hypocritical society that poets and writers constituted an important force opposing "the awakening Hungarians." It is no coincidence that the great poets at the turn of the century had established the most important literary magazine of the time and had called it *Nyugat* (*The West*). They admired Western liberalism and democracy and were inspired in their fight for social and cultural change in the old feudal country.

Poets have played a special role throughout Hungarian history. They have been the real voice of the nation and an essential force against foreign occupation and oppression. The poet Sándor Petőfi fired the opening shot in the 1848 revolution against the Hapsburg Empire when he read his famous inciting poem from the steps of the National Museum in Pest. More than 100 years later, the Hungarian revolt against Russian domination and the Hungarian Stalinists also began with protests by the "Petőfi circle," initially only a small group of poets and writers. Attila, who had died nineteen years earlier, together with Petőfi became symbols of freedom during the 1956 revolution. For the freedom fighters, their words were powerful weapons against tyranny and its opportunistic sycophants. The timelessness of the issue of freedom and its interpretation in Attila's uniquely powerful poetry made his work as relevant and meaningful for the "bourgeoisie and the proletariat," a term he used for his readers. Because he had come to be regarded as such an important symbol of the struggle of freedom against fascist oppression during the 1930s and 1940s, Attila readily became the spokesman for individual freedom in the struggle against Stalinism from 1948 to 1955.

Even today, the sharp contrasts reflected by Attila's poetry seem to be of great relevance. He reflects a confrontation between human rights and the intrinsic order of the countryside, between human needs and the incessant urge of the ruling institution to oversee the activities of its citizens—to control, punish, and persecute. The forms and intensity of such confrontations vary among social systems, but are to be found even in today's most democratic governments, thereby probably reflecting individual opposition against conformity to the state—against becoming an insignificant brick in an enormous edifice. Protests of this sort can be aimed at true oppressors or at scapegoats, those singled out as being responsible for uncontrollable collective industrialization and urbanization. In Attila's world, oppression was a concrete reality, even though the semi-fascist state of Horthy was much less efficient than the totalitarian apparatus to come.

Despite the fact the today's Hungarian youth have grown up in an environment of relatively great freedom of speech, Attila is still highly relevant to them. He is widely read and debated, and he remains a rich subject of essays and research papers. There are many components to this continuing attraction. One essential aspect is the greatness of his poetry, but this alone would not be enough—Hungary has produced a surprisingly large number of great poets. Attila's origins among the poorest of the poor; the resonance that his poetry had for his readers even when he was but a teenager; the complicated involvement with the illegal Communist Party, which resulted in his expulsion; his constant struggle against loneliness and his fear of being ostracized; his insatiable longing for love; and his horrible suicide all contribute to his great appeal. But most important is the content of his poetry. His work reflects the dilemmas confronting the individual in the twentieth century, in which adaptation is often synonymous with a loss of the childish, playful, creative identity.

The playfulness of children is a recurring theme in Attila's writings. The child is a creative creature, able to transcend the limits of everyday routine, rebel against the existing order, and attain true human reality. A child's main activity, play, comes spontaneously from the needs of the personality, without outside direction and "useful" goals. The adult lives within a determined world, his life shaped and decided by outside forces, confined and alone in his "here and now." One of Attila's devoted friends, the author and literary critic Andor Németh, defined the "grown-up" in the image of the young Martin Heidegger:

"Instead of being what he can be to the limits of his available possibilities, the grown up exists as 'one usually does' like all the others, like the 'society,' like a person usually lives." He has fallen into the world where "one" replaces "I." The basic operational concepts are adjustment, indifference, mediocrity, a "normal" existence. The embezzlement of the most essential components of existence will be the price that the adult must pay.

The "well-adjusted" individual in today's highly developed society who feels increasing alienated from our computerized world is just as likely to welcome Attila's message as is the person who is lonely, unloved, and ostracized.

From the dark perspective of his own life, Attila returned repeatedly in his later writings to a utopian "world of freedom," in which the individual can develop and the "handsome and serious son" can live a worthy human life. But this yearning has remained contradictory. "Only I can be my own leader," he wrote. But he was also optimistic about a "free society" that would create conditions in which his thoughts would be tolerated, and in this one can see a logical flaw, more obvious to us today than it could have been for him. A society that permits a degree of freedom far greater than that envisioned by Attila doesn't necessarily promote the nurturing of individuals. The driving force for that, a constant striving for conscious effort and disciplined work, must come from within. Through oppression society can impede, or paradoxically enhance, the development of individuals, but it can never provide a driving force that might be lacking.

Naturally, the issue of "the inner leader" is also a constant and recurring theme in Attila's poetry. Who should provide the commands from within—the intellect, our feelings, or both? If both, in what relation to each other?

Many of Attila's poems start with the phrase "thou shalt." The poet speaks not only to himself but also, at the same time, to someone else. This self-duplication reveals our personal contradictions, in which our intellectual analysis operates in parallel with the world of emotion, revealed as a permanent duality. Nowhere is this polarization more obvious and, in light of Attila's tragic fate, more of an omen than in the poem that Attila wrote on the occasion of Freud's eightieth birthday in 1936, one year before his suicide. At that time he had already been undergoing psychoanalysis for several years. A few sentences from that poem reveal this.

Open for your eyes what you hide in your heart
What you imagine with your eyes, attend it with your heart.
All living creatures are said to die of love, but happiness is vitally
    important, like a piece of bread.
All creatures are children, longing for a mother's womb.
If you don't embrace, you kill. The battlefield is a nuptial bed.
Thou shalt be like the embattled octagenarian, who begets millions
    of new sons while bleeding.
The thorn that got stuck in the sole of your foot long ago has long
    since vanished.
Your own death will fall out of your heart soundlessly, soon.
Grab what you imagine with your eyes, embrace or kill the one you
    love! [13]

The opening lines reflect Attila's underlying analytical approach. Inner reality is elevated to the surface, although it is still necessary to search for its subjective meaning. The emotional content of concrete observations can come to light only after patient waiting. The connection between love and death, Eros and Thanatos, are a reflection of the Freudian dialectic. The individual dissolves into another being, gives up his own self and dies, even as he confirms his own self. The bliss of love is as essential as the bread of life. In his double exhortation to the reader and to himself, the poet proposes an identification with the eighty-year-old Freud, the father, who is constantly subjected to the aggressions of his sons but who continues to transform this world. The poet is filled with admiration for the father of what he still hopes is a redeeming analytical method. Freud is portrayed in an aura of almost divine splendor and in an unwavering state of balance between antipodes of destruction and resurrection. But the status of the writer-patient is also intertwined with this image, unobtrusively and silently. The thorn, stuck for such a long time in the sole, is suddenly gone, but soon his own death will also fall silently and unnoticeably from his heart. This becomes a recurring motif for Attila's late poems. The following year, in his last poem written just days before his suicide, he says, "Now even my death is useless." Was he later to insert his head and arms between the railroad carriages to regain that lost meaning of his death?

The analytical process is also expressed in many other poems from Attila's later period, and the relationship of a mother and son is a central focus. His abandoned mother was forced to leave the three-year-old Attila and his sisters with the family of an unknown farmer, leaving incurable scars in Attila. When they were finally reunited four years later, she was completely exhausted and had no time or strength for her children. Incessant troubles, coldness, and starvation were the unremitting themes, and the abysmal deprivation left Attila with an insatiable yearning for love as an adult. He continuously sought out his mother in his mind and in his poetry, but through psychotherapy he came to realize that her sainted image existed only in his fantasy world. He searched in vain for his dead mother in all of his love relationships; this unfulfilled yearning undermined his self-confidence and left him ever more bitter and isolated.

All agreed, even Attila, that he put impossible demands on the women he loved. In one of his last and most wonderful poems, he writes in his unique and untranslatable language:

If you don't press me to your bosom
like your only possession
while you are dreaming and laughing in your sleep,
the thieves will snatch me away
and then you will recline on the sofa, crying
what an orphan and how foolish I am.

If you don't tell me, every minute,
that you are happy, because you live for me,
you can chat to your bowing shadow
when loneliness and fear torment you.
You won't have a line to strengthen your love
if it becomes totally threadbare.

If you don't make love devouring me,
trees, hills and waves will batter me.
I love you, like a child would love,
and I am as cruel as he is.
I will darken the hall where you
bathe in light. I'll die.

Attila's Illness and Death

Over the half century since his death, the last two years of Attila's life have continued to fascinate the Hungarian public and have stimulated numerous studies and commentaries by psychologists, psychiatrists, literary historians, poets, and other writers. The public has come to regard him with greater respect than any other modern writer. His illness and death have been viewed from strongly polarized perspectives, but his literary greatness has never been subject to dispute.

According to the earlier, generally accepted view, Attila suffered from a serious mental illness. The psychiatrist who treated him during his last year, Dr. Robert Bak, made the diagnosis of schizophrenia and thought that he could trace the slow onset of the disorder to poetry written when Attila was still a teenager. He also pointed to Attila's repeated attempts at suicide as further evidence of schizophrenia.

Attila himself has described how, at the age of eighteen, he tried for the third time to kill himself by lying on the railroad tracks. He waited for the train to run him over, but it never arrived. After a while, he stood up and walked along the tracks to try to find out what had gone wrong. It became apparent that the train had hit someone else committing suicide farther up the tracks. Attila often referred to this incident in his letters. Trains certainly played a major role in Attila's fantasy world, and the train theme recurred repeatedly in his writings. It was therefore hardly a coincidence that his life came to a close under a train.

Dr. Bak, who emigrated to the United States after the war, published and successively revised several clinical descriptions of Attila's illness, from childhood to his death. Some of his interpretations are astonishing to today's reader. Most of this century's great poets might just as easily be labeled mentally ill on similar grounds. Attila's subtle and refined sensitivity, his unique language, and the richness of his symbolism are derived directly from the world of childhood and dreams, and their daring contrasts have a stunning impact on the modern reader. These same qualities, however, were seen by the cultural conservatives of his time to be pathological symptoms of illness. The following episode illustrates one such misunderstanding.

Robert Bak and later writers have quoted from a poem that they claim gives evidence of "pathological sensations from the internal organs of the body, typical symptoms of progressive schizophrenia." They pointed particularly to the following lines: "Do not start any mischief in my intestines, do not knock in my chest, do not throw away my bean-shaped kidneys."

Attila's friend, the psychiatrist István Kulcsár, later pointed out that Attila at that time was reading the Finnish saga *Kalevala* every day, and that the poem was written in the same rhythm as *Kalevala*. In the seventeenth runo (canto) of *Kalevala,* the giant Vipuinen swallows Väinämöinen, causing him violent abdominal pain. In words similar to those of Attila's poem, he begs his unwelcome guest to "quit my liver, let my heart be undevoured, leave thou, too, my spleen uninjured."[14]

All the descriptions of Attila's illness have attached great importance to the psychoanalysis he undertook six years before his death. His companion from 1930 to 1936, Judit Szántó, described Attila's encounter with his first psychoanalyst, Samuel Rapaport, on tram line six in 1931.[15] Attila knew Rapaport from his student days in Szeged, and they were very happy to meet again. Rapaport wanted to give Attila a job and asked him to come for a visit. As usual, Attila was broke and therefore gladly accepted the task, to proofread Rapaport's book, *Origin and Treatment of Nervous Stomach and Intestinal Disorders.* Attila carried out the job with great care and became familiar with many disorders of the stomach and intestines. According to Judit, Attila discovered one symptom after another in himself as he proceeded with the work. Some six months before his meeting with Rapaport, Attila and Judit had gone to a doctor for his stomach troubles, which he was told resulted from prolonged starvation during his childhood and the state of malnutrition evident at the time of his visit to the doctor. Starvation is a constantly recurring theme in Attila's writings. He had always been very thin, and his sisters worried about his diet.

Attila refused to charge Rapaport anything for his work, asking instead that the psychiatrist accept him for analysis. Rapaport hesitated at first, but finally agreed to take on Attila as a patient. Attila was obviously seeking help, but he was also interested in learning more about the analytical method and its reputed potential for providing a more profound understanding of oneself and the human condition.[16] It is not completely clear at what point the purpose of the sessions changed from training to patient analysis. However, as early as 1934 Attila wrote that "a sick world is trying to foist its unacceptably pathological views upon me so as to eventually classify me as sick. I am getting into an untenable situation."

Attila had every reason to consider his world of 1934 to be hopelessly sick. The youthful revolutionary who represented the poor and oppressed, the socialist who believed more in his own innate and profoundly humane ideas than in the authority and discipline of the Communist Party, was ostracized by the illegal and harshly centralized Party. The process began when Attila was not selected as a delegate to a literary congress in Moscow and ended in his expulsion from the Party in 1934. The official and semi-official ideologues of the various communist regimes in Hungary always found it difficult to explain these events, because they invariably regarded Attila as the greatest revolutionary poet since Sandor Petőfi and Endre Ady.

The expulsion was a particularly harsh blow to Attila. He was deprived of membership in the only established group to which he had ever belonged, and he also lost some of his closest friends. But Attila had no choice. He could not possibly accept the sham show trials of Stalinism, to which he referred as "fascist communism." Stalinism thoroughly destroyed all hope for a more humane society, exactly as the onslaught of Hitler's Third Reich had done.

It is difficult to identify the exact moment at which word of Attila's mental instability began to circulate among his friends and acquaintances. He always discussed his problems and his analysis quite openly with his friends. He certainly had a deep personal interest in the process of analysis, but he also entered into his own treatments with exaggerated expectations. Rapaport was apparently unable to deal successfully with the enormous complex of experiences and problems that underlay Attila's symptoms. He began to think that Attila suffered from early schizophrenia and told others of his diagnosis. His goal was to stabilize his patient's condition and prevent it from deteriorating. But he told the poet that he had a severe form of neurasthenia and involved him in the concepts of his analysis. Attila realized that something was not quite right. He wrote, "One pulls me here, another jerks me there. Everyone grabs at me, babbling and pushing, but no one pays attention to my hunchback."

During his analysis, Attila's guilt feelings were continually reinforced, and he was unable to attain a state of serenity and reconciliation. Childhood experiences and repressed sexual episodes came to the surface. In vain, Attila searched his soul for forgiveness and deliverance. Failing in that, he tried to find relief from his symptoms and liberate himself from the labels that became attached to him.

In the early part of 1935, Rapaport concluded that he could not continue the analysis. After several unsuccessful intermediary attempts, Attila was referred to a woman analyst, Edith Gyömröi. He attended sessions with her for two years, but they seemed to have a very detrimental effect on him. In 1936 Attila's emotional attachment, a natural feeling of a patient toward his analyst, turned into a fervent love that remained completely unrequited. The erotic transformation of the patient's feelings endangered everything the analyst had hoped to achieve. There was an insoluble conflict between Attila's unlimited need for maternal love and any chances he might have had for achieving an understanding of his problems. Edith Gyömröi became aware of the problem after it was already too late to change matters and only after Attila had become unmanageable. She discontinued the therapy, declaring that he was no longer suited for analysis.

Attila's friends who were aware of only half the story must have concluded that he was desperately ill. Again, the poet reexperienced the childhood loss of his mother. His feeling that he was undeserving of love was confirmed, and he was dealt an additional serious blow to his self-confidence as a man.

None of this had any effect on the poet's creativity. Some of his most beautiful works were written during this period. The poems from the early part of the analysis with Gyömröi express a feeling of happy and self-redeeming love, like the unsuspicious and assured exuberant love of a child longing for its mother. His total devotion is reflected in this poem:

You Made Me Child

You made me child, why agony for thirty years?
I cannot walk and I cannot sit here helpless.
My legs jolt me in your direction.

I hold you in my mouth like a dog his pup,
and I would run to keep from choking on you.
The years that shattered my life
break on me every moment.

Feed me. I am hungry, cover me, I am cold.
I am regressed. Give me your attention.
Your absence penetrates like a draft in the house.
Command fear to leave me.
You looked at me and I forgot everything.
You listened and my speech stuck.
Make me exorable.
Teach me how to live and die alone.
My mother threw me out and I lie out of doors
where I want to hide in myself but where is it?
Beneath me stone and above an emptiness.
I would like to sleep. I knock at your house.

There are many who are unfeeling like me
and still they cry.
I love for I learned to love myself with you.[17]

But in a few short months, other sounds are heard:

Afraid to Love

You prostitute who fears love
and prizes the security of work
the aphid heavens string on our neck

sending the eternal freeze so early—
inverted whore, you accumulate
obligations under an open sky—
a child may whine for love
but I cannot help it. I must do away with you.[18]

The culmination is reached in his poem of hate, "Loneliness."
Has a more beautiful poem of hate ever been written?

A bug crawls on your open eyes. Green
mold cover your breast with down.
Look into the loneliness where you send me.
Grind your molars and swallow your tongue.

Let your face blow like dry sand,
and when you want to pet
because of emptiness in your lap
let a weed entangle your hand.

You are an ugly desire
and would not even blink
if they silently sat around and watched
who turned me into such a fiend.

Whom are you clasping now? Give birth
and your son will play ring-a-rose
while you peek, and full-fed alligators
slither about on their bellies.

I lie motionless in bed.
I see my Eye—you eavesdrop with it.
Die! I want it so much
I could die for it.[19]

Attila's aggression took form not only in artistic expression but
also in very concrete threats. Gyömröi came to the definite
conclusion that Attila was suffering from a psychosis and turned
the treatment over to the psychiatrist Robert Bak, who continued
the sessions until the poet's death. At this time, one year before
his suicide, the vicious circle of stigmatization was already in full
swing. What had previously been interpreted as signs of extraordinary sensitivity, a remarkable ability to think along several paths
simultaneously and contrast several different realities, now came
to be interpreted as symptoms of pathology. The poetry of Attila's
last year revealed an increasing alienation and exclusion from
contact with others and a blurred border between illness and

health. His correspondence and notes from this period to friends and relatives bear witness to an increasingly indistinct tangle of facts and delusions. Attila's change of analysts should have been respected as a private matter, but it was not. It created a stir in numerous circles and was considered almost a matter of public interest. Attila's return to a normal life therefore became even more difficult. Robert Bak took this as confirmation that Attila was mentally ill and, from all appearances, he said as much directly or indirectly even to Attila's relatives and friends. The reaction of friends and colleagues varied from rejection to compassion, from a desire to "help the sick back to the world of the normal" to a persistent anxiety over the possibility that "anything can happen, anytime." But the most important effect, and probably the most damaging, was the fact that Attila was no longer being taken seriously. His poetry was still admired, but he was greeted in the course of everyday life with a superficiality and indifference usually reserved for those considered "completely mad."

Dr. Bak was convinced that Attila was not a suitable patient for analysis, but he wanted to avoid the usual consequence that would have followed his diagnosis, that is, institutionalization in a mental hospital. In contrast to the professional standards of the time, he decided to proceed with psychiatric treatment in his own office. His "therapy" consisted mainly of friendly personal conversations—attempts to show understanding, to reassure, and "to hope for a miracle." Attila called his writings from this period "bubbles from my anguished soul." They reflect an increasingly desperate yearning for deep and devoted love, for human contact, and for peace. Instead he found only indecision, anguish, and real or imaginary hostility. The medical and paramedical people in charge of his care struggled for a clearer understanding of his illness and for a better-defined program of treatment. However, all their efforts were futile and only strengthened their feelings of uncertainty and ambivalence. Attila interpreted this attitude as yet another rejection, but this time it was in the context of a truly desperate situation in which he needed resoluteness and support. The attempts at treatment thereby merely aggravated his illness. They even had deleterious effects on the poet's relatives and friends. They were given "expert" explanations of his behav-

ior, descriptions of the mysterious border line between normality
and illness that they accepted respectfully. But with that they also
distanced themselves from him, looking upon him as a sick man
whose illness had begun silently and secretly in the distant past.

At the beginning of 1937, Attila tried desperately to become
involved in a new love affair. His letters to Flóra Kozmucza, to
whom he dedicated some of his most beautiful poems, reveal,
however, a certain feeling of distance. We will return to this later.
Flóra tried to hold out "hope for a miracle" rather than giving him
the unreserved love he needed. When Flóra became ill herself
and went away for treatment in July 1937, Attila broke down. He
was treated in a private nursing home for several months before
his two sisters invited him to come to their home near Lake
Balaton. It was there that he spent the last months of his life and
where he killed himself on December 3, 1937.

Attila's poetry from the last year of his life shows no weakening
of his artistic inspiration. His astounding choice of words and the
structure of his language that had captivated his readers through
the years remained as masterful and full of surprises as before.
In contrast to Dr. Bak's theory that Attila's illness had progressed
inexorably, some contemporary and more recent observers have
pointed out that his writing was at its artistic and intellectual peak,
which is quite obvious to the Hungarian-speaking reader. Not
even the poems he wrote during his last week showed any significant signs of mental disturbance, except for his increasingly
desperate cries for friendship stemming from his deepening
isolation. His last poem ends with a quiet sense of resignation.

I Finally Found My Home

I finally found my home
the land where my name
is correctly spelled above the grave
where I'm buried—if I'm buried.

This earth will take me in
like an alms box.
No one wants a worthless coin
left over from the days of war,

or the iron ring engraved with
the fine words: new world, rights,
land. Our laws are still for war
and gold rings are preferred.

I was alone for a long time.
Then many came to visit me.
'You live alone' they said, though
gladly I would have lived among them.

That's how I lived, in vain,
I'll be the first to say.
They made me play the fool.
Now even my death is useless.

While I lived, I tried
to stand up against the whirlwind.
The joke is, I harmed less
than I was harmed.

Spring is fine, and so is summer,
but autumn's better and winter's best
for one who finally leaves his hopes
for a family and a home to others.[20]

Word for word, the last sentence in the original Hungarian
means ". . .but winter is the most beautiful season for one who
can hope for home and hearth now only for the sake of others."

In his descriptions of the case history, Dr. Bak tried to resolve
the discrepancy between the patient's clarity of logic and his own
unequivocal diagnosis by making a distinction between the poet
whose artistic talents were unaffected by the illness and the
desperately sick man himself. He described the "pathological"
manifestations hiding behind the purely artistic expressions. He
praised the wonderful grasp of the poetry on abstract reality, but
considered Attila's absence of contact with true reality to be a
pathological expression of his self-absorption and separation
from human contact, resulting in isolation, ambivalence, aggression, exaggerated attachment, the need for love, incomprehensible thought associations, anguish, and fear.

In a rather self-righteous summary of the case history, Dr. Bak
wrote that one could "with a certain assurance conclude that
Attila was still able to remain a poet even when he was so seriously
mentally deranged." It has been pointed out by Bókay, Jádi, and
Stark that this wording tends to absolve both Dr. Bak and his
patient from all responsibility for the events of his life. Of course,
Attila is not to blame—his illness is at fault. Likewise, if Attila is
not responsible for the inexorable course of events, then no one
else is answerable for it either.

Three Thirty-Two-Year-Olds Suggest an Alternative Interpretation

Three thirty-two-year-old Hungarian writers, A. Bókay, F. Jádi, and A. Stark, have formulated a different interpretation of Attila's illness, based on the reports of Dr. Bak and other contemporary commentators as well as on their own analyses of Attila's work. According to them, the first determining step was taken by Attila himself during his adolescence, when he distanced himself from his fellow human beings and chose norms of behavior different from those of the majority. This movement received its first great artistic expression in the poem "Innocent Song," the work that resulted in his expulsion from training for a teaching career. In this poem, with the innocent and fresh spirit of a twenty-year-old, Attila rejected the four basic pillars of society: father, mother, God, and country. The reaction of Professor Horger was typical for that time and carried with it a clear symbolic message. Horger took it upon himself to deny the young revolutionary the benefits of society to which he considered only the socially well-adjusted entitled. These harsh measures made it impossible for Attila to adjust and made his break with society irrevocable. But Dr. Bak interpreted the episode in a completely different way. He considered it to be the first manifestation of an incipient mental illness that was parallelled by a "progressive narrowing" of the circle to which Attila wished to belong.

Naturally, Attila sought out like-minded people. At first he thought he had found them in the underground Communist Party, and for a short time he devoted himself intensely to that cause. But Bak considered even that a bad omen. He believed Attila's attraction to the extreme political left to have been a manifestation of latent aggression and an inability to establish close human contacts. Politically conservative himself, Bak considered it "an instinctively determined attempt to conceal an inability for emotionally mature personal contacts behind the facade of a collective involvement."

Attila's membership in the Communist Party was anything but a sign of self- assertion or an expression of latent aggression. Several commentators have emphasized that his activities in the Party were quite rational and constructive. His expulsion from the Party was therefore especially tragic because it kept him from filling the void left by his previous rejection by the established society. He had only one alternative left—to build his identity through the strength of his own inner resources—but even that was made impossible by the stigmatization caused by his illness. There was no longer any question of exclusion from a particular social or political group, but rather of a separation from the entire world of human beings.

Attila's stigmatization took on a particularly gruesome form during the fall of 1937, when the social democratic newspaper *Népszava* published an article entitled "Attila József's Illness." The paper's editors apparently thought it appropriate to inform their readers about the poet's nursing-home treatment for a nervous breakdown. Attila was completely distraught when he learned of the article: "Now everyone knows I am crazy." His sense of utter isolation was further reinforced when his colleagues stopped referring him for editorial work for a literary magazine. These former colleagues showed clearly that they had lost confidence in him, withholding information they had previously shared.

Attila realized that he could not construct an accurate sense of reality from the remaining shattered fragments with which he had contact. The drastic therapy he had been given, including insulin shock treatments, had only made his condition worse. Because of that, his physician and supporters abandoned any thoughts of continued hospitalization. They tried to convince Attila that the treatments had worked, and they discharged him with instructions to resume his writing. But Attila took that as an admission that they had all given up on him, and that no one was able to help him any longer. In his letters to Flóra, he wrote that he did not feel secure anywhere, he had lost all sense of human worth, and he felt that no one liked him. He felt "ugly, weak, and a nobody," and unworthy of Flóra. He suffered from tormenting feelings of guilt and felt persecuted for imaginary and ill-defined crimes.

In Dr. Bak's published report, this entire process is described as a further indication of the progression of his mental illness. But the three thirty-two-year-olds indicate, not without bitterness, that a similar judgment could be passed on many of the other poets of the twentieth century.

Dr. Bak selected certain later poems to illustrate his hypothesis of a rapidly progressing mental illness. But even these poems can be taken as expressions of Attila's fear that the diagnosis of his illness might become true. "Don't be harsh with me if I become mad. Just hold me back with your strong arms," he wrote. The same vision of the dreaded mental disease is expressed in the remarkable line, "When I come to squint with my entire being." Bak took this as evidence for the "bizarre images" induced by the pressure of his illness. But in Attila's poetry, the phrase is more brilliant than bizarre.

Schizophrenia in poets is often revealed through a decomposition of verse construction and an increasingly meaningless jumble of words. That never occurs in Attila's writing. On the contrary, his style shows a progressive and classical process of literary maturation, increased precision, and growing clarity. There is no evidence of pathological confusion, the three authors point out. Attila's is a healthy eye looking at a pathological world. It was Dr. Bak who saw evidence of mental illness in the views expressed in Attila's poetry, and by doing so, he torpedoed Attila's struggle to regain his health.

Szárszó, a small village near Lake Balaton, was to become Attila's last stop in life. It was there, in the care of his two sisters, that he was supposed to rest but where, in the dreary gray and cold autumn, he experienced his most complete disassociation from the world. In one of his last poems, he wrote:

I am vanquished (if there is victory)
but whom do I surrender to?
I fell from every other world
like fruit from a tree.
The learned doctors inject me, shield me,
and "I work"—look at all this paper.
They write to me, I read.
I find my rest in keeping busy.
Without you who play with me,
I would be an animal and shameless.
Among you I went crazy, I the finite.
I am a human being, and hence ridiculous.[21]

His longing for death and its fulfillment in his suicide was the only logical outcome. The three authors write of his presuicidal symptoms; his increasing tendency to screen himself off from all contacts with the world; his obsession with one distant person, Flóra; and the gruesome and and almost inexorable "plot" that led finally to his suicide. Everyone took part in this plot: the poet himself, his relatives and friends, his doctors, and the whole of society that knew him and his work. In a subconscious and reluctant sort of way, they all contributed to the inevitable message to Attila: "It's probably best if you were to die." The literary public was able to retain its idolized poet only by sacrificing the man. Only one of Attila's colleagues, Zsigmond Reményik, dared to formulate these thoughts, in the periodical *Szép Szó* (*The Beautiful Word*). He emphasized that the social stigmatization had an irreversible effect on Attila. If Attila had survived, he would have always been confronted by "unsympathetic slander and distortion," and "only through his death was Attila able to escape his future so badly gone astray."

Attila's sisters have described the events of his last days, especially in the book by Jolán József. They followed the doctors' orders and kept their brother under constant supervision, ready for the mental illness expected to erupt at any moment. They didn't allow him to go anywhere alone, and he was constantly surrounded by his own private mental institution. Now and then he made some efforts to resist by refusing to get off the train, refusing to eat, or denying that he had any medical problems whatsoever and was merely trying to become a mature, healthy poet. At other times he was able to discuss, quite matter-of-factly, that he had only two alternatives: to marry Flóra and return to literary activities, or commit suicide. The first seemed paradoxical—if he accepted the stigma of his illness, the only thing that had kept him alive, the message inherent in his writing, would lose all its validity. He also knew that Flóra considered him seriously ill, which is why she had told him to stay where he was and wait for a miracle.

The sisters were obviously not able to provide any significant support for Attila. They hid his razor blades, they were concerned when he gazed at the express trains speeding by, and they feared that he would jump into the well or drown himself in the bathtub. Attila's last "cry for help," to use the psychiatric terminology, came the day before his suicide. Some friends and colleagues came for a visit, and Attila seemed happy in their company. As they prepared to set off for their return trip to Budapest, Attila asked if he could join them. "No, there wasn't enough room in the car. You can come to see us next week." Attila begged them time and again, even as they were standing next to the car about to leave. They managed to convince him only by demonstrating how crowded the car was: there were five people in a car designed for four. It would be impossible to squeeze in even a small dog, let alone a sixth person. The three authors comment that Attila probably detected a frightful symbolism in that remark: "There is no place for you in this world, even if you were to shrink to the size of a little dog." That is how it must have sounded to him. One day later, he commited suicide at the very spot where he took his leave from the car. For years afterward, many other people, most of them young, followed in Attila's footsteps at that exact spot. It has taken on a gruesome and almost cultlike significance.

The course of events during the day of his suicide give the impression of deliberate and careful preparation. Attila said goodbye in four short but lucid letters, mailing them with no apparent concern. To Dr. Bak he wrote, "I send you my warmest greetings. In vain you have tried the impossible." He embraced his sister Jolán intensely, and although she did not realize it, that embrace was his goodbye to her. The sisters knew nothing about the letters until after they were delivered.

The Three Women

Three women who were close to the poet during different periods in his life have published their memoirs. Flóra was the object of Attila's last great love, or rather a budding, tentative love that inspired many of his great poems during the last six months of his life. It was only quite recently that Professor Flóra Kozmucza, widow of the poet Gyula Illyés, succumbed to the relentless curiosity and the legend surrounding Attila by publishing a small memoir.[22] The young psychologist Flóra met Attila for the first time on February 20, 1937, nine months before his suicide. That meeting took place in the home of one of her friends, who had invited some writers and psychologists to visit. Attila was taken there by one of his writer friends who wanted Flóra to perform a Rorschach analysis on him. Flóra loved poetry, and so she paid more attention to Attila than to most other patients. She was captivated by Attila's sympathetic and restless personality, although he did not really appeal to her as a man. She performed only about half of the Rorschach test, and never completed it. The test results appeared bizarre and very unusual to Flora. But Attila grew weary of the test in the middle and continued half-heartedly, "only for Flórá's sake," as he said.

The results of the test have never been made public, but according to Flórá's book, they revealed some "rather unusual symptoms" that would not have been anticipated from his behavior or from his poetry. But she hastens to point out that one must not reach any conclusions from only one test, and certainly far less from only half a test.

After a little while, Flóra and Attila interrupted the test and Attila went on to recite some of his poems. Everyone gathered around and listened with rapt attention. One of the poems was called "Tante Lidi" (quoted at the beginning of this essay). The other, "Ode," is one of Attila's greatest works.

Ode

1.

I am sitting
here on a glittering wall of rocks.
The mellow wind of the young summer
like the warmth of a good supper
flies around.

I let my heart grow fond of silence.
It is not so difficult,
—the past swarms around—
the head bends down
and down hangs the hand.

I gaze at the mountain's mane
every leaf reflects the glow
of your brow.
The road is empty, empty,
yet I can see
how the wind makes your skirt flutter
under the fragile branches of the tree.
I see a lock of your hair tip forward
your soft breasts quiver
—as the stream down below is running away—

behold, I see again,
how the ripples on round white pebbles
the fairy laughter spouts out on your teeth.

2.

O how I love you
who, made to speak
both, the wily solitude which weaves its plots
in the deepest caverns of the heart
and the universe.
Who, part from me, in silence, and run away
like the waterfall from its own rumble
while I, between the peaks of my life,
near to the far,
cry out and reverberate
rebounding against sky and earth
that I love you, you sweet step-mother.

3.

I love you like the child loves his mother,
like silent pits love their depth
I love you like halls love the light
like the soul loves the flame,
like the body loves repose.
I love you like all mortals love living
until they die.

Every single smile, movement, word of yours
I keep like the earth keeps all fallen matter.
Like acids into metal
so my instincts have burnt
your dear and beautiful form into my mind,
and there your being fills up everything.

Moments pass by, rattling
but you are sitting mutely in my ears.
Stars blaze and fall
but you stand still in my eyes.
Like silence in a cave,
your flavour, now cool
still lingers in my mouth
and your hand upon the waterglass
and the delicate veins upon your hand
glimmer up before me again and again.

4.

O what kind of matter am I
that your glance cuts and shapes me?
What kind of soul and what kind of light

and what kind of amazing phenomenon am I
that in the mist of emptiness
I can walk around
the gentle slopes of your fertile body?

And like the word
entering into an enlightened mind
I can enter into its mysteries.

Your veins like rosebushes
tremble ceaselessly.
They carry the eternal current
that love may blossom in your cheeks
and thy womb may bear a blessed fruit.

Many a small root embroiders through and through
the sensitive soil of your stomach
weaving knots, unwinding the tangle
that the cells of your juices may align
into clusters of swarming lines
and that the good thickets of your bushy lungs
may whisper their own glory.

The eternal matter happily proceeds in you
along the tunnels of your bowels
and the waste gains a rich life
in the hot wells of your ardent kidneys.

Undulating hills rise
star constellations oscillate
lakes move, factories operate
millions of living creatures
insects
seaweed
cruelty and goodness stir
the sun shines, a misty arctic light looms—
unconscious eternity roams about
in your metabolism.

5.

Like clots of blood
these words fall
before you.
Existence stutters
only the law speaks clearly.
But my industrious organs that renew me
day by day
are now preparing for silence.

But until then all cry out.
You,

whom they have selected out of the multitude
of two thousand million people,
you only one,
you soft cradle,
strong grave, living bed
receive me into you!...

(How tall is the sky at dawn!
Armies are dazzling in its ore.
This great radiance hurts my eyes.
I am lost, I believe...
I hear my heart beating
Flapping above me.)

6.

(By-song.)

(The train is taking me, I am going
perhaps I may even find you today.
My burning face may then cool down,
and perhaps you will softly say:

The water is running, take a bath.
Here is a towel for you to dry.
The meat is cooking, appease your hunger,
this is your bed, where I lie.)[23]

Promptly the next day, Attila phoned Flóra at her office, a
gesture that was considered most unusual and even improper by
the head of her institute. Attila asked to see her for an important
conversation, but she was very busy. In addition to a crowded work
schedule, Flóra also supported herself by giving private French
lessons in the evenings. They were not able to meet until three
days later, at a café. As a gift, Attila gave her a big bundle of poems,
love poems written during those three days. Flóra, whose name
appeared everywhere in the poems, was touched and flattered,
but she could not identify with the Flóra in the poems. The writing
was very beautiful and earnest, but aimed at a different person,
one she did not recognize. But she was deeply moved when she
realized what a "stormy feeling" had been aroused in Attila during
such a short period of time. She later came to understand that
his feelings were rooted much more deeply than merely in their
short and casual acquaintance. Attila seemed to be searching for
a sanctuary, a place where he could hide from his own disappointments and from his incurable deprivation of parental love. Dur-

ing the very first hour of their first private conversation, Attila asked Flóra if she would marry him.

Flóra was both moved and frightened by his words, his passionate sensitivity, and his earnestness. She felt a deep sympathy for this combination of enormous talent and immense suffering. She was amazed by the simultaneous presence of chaos and rigorously disciplined logic. But most of all, she was entranced by the aura surrounding him—an aura, of all things, of unending playfulness and delight. But at the same time, she instinctively felt that she ought not see him any more. But by then it was too late.

Their meetings during the spring of 1937 were squeezed into Florá's tight schedule, often after Attila had waited patiently for her. They went for long walks and enjoyed conversations in cafés. Flóra writes in her book that there was never any sexual relationship between them, as unbelievable as that might sound to today's youth. But sexual relationships were quite unthinkable among properly brought-up middle-class girls of that time.

The many relaxed springtime walks ended suddenly when Flóra was afflicted with a severe heart ailment. After her hospitalization and during her convalescence in the Mátra mountains, she and Attila corresponded. She suggested that he come to visit her, but for some reason that she had trouble understanding in retrospect, the visit never took place. Did Attila doubt his own feelings? Was it that his "inner golden scale," which according to his friend and colleague Lörinc Szabó could detect the slightest movements of even lights and shadows, was able to feel Florá's uncertainty?

When Flóra returned to Budapest, Attila was already under treatment at the nursing home "Siesta." Their correspondence that followed leaves a frightening impression. The combination of shock and drug treatment had a marked effect on Attila. His letters were often confusing and incoherent, and Attila was fully aware of it. He begged incessantly for Flóra to visit him, but for prolonged periods his doctors didn't permit her to come. On one occasion she went to Budapest, but was not allowed to see Attila. Their correspondence swung from cheerful plans for the future, and even of marriage, to the darkest desperation.

During the fall of 1937, Flóra was finally granted permission to visit Attila on a regular basis. By then, however, he had become very unstable, and he was often in a dark mood and broke down into sobbing spells as the time came to separate. He became suspicious and jealous, and found it difficult to trust Flóra. It was not possible for him to maintain any feelings of optimism from one day to another. On occasion he became quite aggressive, once even choking Flóra until all went black before her eyes. The scene was interrupted only when a nurse came into the room.

Flóra paints a grim picture of Attila's last weeks near Lake Balaton, but it is difficult to know how much of her description corresponds to reality. Her book was written several decades later and only after the questions and accusations of a number of generations. But it is quite clear that Flóra, like Attila's other friends, had more or less come to accept her friend's illness, and that he sat there alone and isolated in the darkness of that November. She visited him one week before his death, and brought apples for his sister's children. They agreed that she would return the following Sunday.

In his short farewell letter to Flóra, Attila wrote:

Dear Flóra:
Forgive me. I do believe in miracles. But for me, there exists only one miracle, and I will carry it out. The rest didn't depend on us . . . I kiss your hand and send my greetings with great friendship and love. We thank you for the apples. I also ate some, although they were meant for the children and I didn't even ask for permission to take some.
Attila
P.S. Please do not come next Sunday.

Judit Szántó also published her memoirs about Attila, together with other parts of her diary. Her book was published posthumously. She was Attila's constant companion and lived with him from 1930 to 1936. Like Attila, Judit came from a harsh and deprived proletarian background, and she had also been very active in the illegal communist movement. Even at the beginning of her book, she paints a picture of a devoted party member straddling the line between dogmatism and fanaticism. That was also true of Attila at the beginning of their relationship, but he lacked her sense of dogmatism, which proved to be a source of conflict between them. Judit complains frequently about Attila's tendency to provoke a discussion and immediately take the opposite view of his interlocutor, whatever it was. She found this repulsive. According to her, Attila used to espouse extreme left-wing views when he was exposed to right-wing people, but when talking to communists, he would act more like a conservative. "Say something, and I will tear your argument apart," was his favorite reply. According to Judit, it is therefore no surprise that Attila, who needed friendship more than anyone else, lost friends so easily.

Apart from that point, her book does not provide any penetrating insights into Attila, but it does present a picture of their often stormy relationship. Judit's writing is very emotional, oscillating between love and hate and often becoming sentimental. If one didn't already know a great deal about Attila, it would be very difficult to discern the poet behind her unsettled writing, so filled with accusations and feelings of aggression, guilt, and prejudice. Now and then she calls Attila "my poor little thing" and looks upon him as if he were a weeping, insecure little boy, unable to take care of himself or his business affairs, always in debt and no better off than a beggar with his hand constantly stretched out for a loan. She accuses him of lacking courage and too readily yielding his political principles, especially in his relationship with Baron Hatvany, his patron and protector. "He allows himself to be bribed with a piece of bread," she declares, using an old Hungarian phrase. But Judit's strongest attacks are directed at Attila's circle of friends. It is known from other sources that many of his friends regarded her as a destructive force in Attila's life, or at least, certainly not the life companion the poet needed. At best, they saw her as the tool for the fulfillment of Attila's sexual needs. One of Attila's closest friends, the author Zsigmond Reményik, wrote that Judit destroyed Attila's self-confidence by humiliating him frequently in front of his friends.

There are only a few places in which her story takes on a more serious tone, where the reader might detect something of the more positive characteristics that must have contributed to her power of attraction over the young Attila. That seems to happen often in political contexts. In response to the rise of Nazism, she expressed a deep concern for the future of socialism and for humanity itself. She was afraid that the disintegrating working class would be so taken in or intoxicated by "the colorful, gaudy rags" of fascism that it would turn self-destructively against its own principles and interests.

Judit had every reason to worry. Her daughter from her first marriage, Eva, fled to the Soviet Union with her father in the 1930s. The father had been closely connected with Béla Kun, the leader of the Hungarian communist regime in 1919 that was ousted from power after only several months. He was a member of the small clique of communist emigrants around Kun in Moscow, and he eventually married Kun's daughter. Judit didn't hear from her daughter for many years, and her book reflects all the torment that a mother can feel for an only daughter of whose fate she knows nothing. The situation was further complicated when she learned that her former husband, whom she still respected, was put on trial together with Kun himself. Kun was eventually executed during the Stalin purges of 1939.

Judit's daughter survived and returned to Hungary at the end of the war, only to commit suicide herself. Except for the many personal problems, these human destinies are all characterized by an emotion often described but seldom well articulated in Judit's book—a disappointment in "the God that failed," to use Arthur Koestler's words. She was appalled by the degeneration of Stalinist socialism. Ambivalence runs like a red thread through the fabric of Judit's book. She throws herself abruptly between her undiminished admiration for the Soviet Union, her "real homeland," and her misgivings about the Stalinist society, in which she noticed that "no one helps another human being." Judit's book gives a vivid account of the tragedy of European communism during the 1930s. The committed and idealistic communists among her closest friends had wagered everything on the Party and believed in the USSR with the intensity of a religious faith. They dismissed as bourgeois propaganda all the negative rumors of what was happening in the Soviet Union.

One of Judit's friends from her work and from the Party was none other than János Kádár, who was later to write that Judit was a skillful agitator. During breaks in her work, she often used to read aloud the letters from her daughter Eva, describing her wonderful life in Moscow. Eva wrote that she was taking piano lessons and that the family was planning a vacation trip to the Crimea.

But quite abruptly, her daughter's letters stopped coming. Judit went to the Soviet embassy to try to get some information, but in vain. She listened to the Hungarian-language broadcasts from Radio Moscow, wondering whether something like this could possibly happen, if there could be any truth to what the conservative newspapers were reporting, but quickly rejecting those thoughts as mere hostile propaganda against the working class. Her writing moves from faith and hope to despair and anguish. She felt just as trapped as Attila, but unlike him, she was unable to free herself from her attachment to the Party. Like many others in the Party, she was caught up in its ideology, inspired partly through her own convictions and partly through a defiance of the Nazi persecutions, only to discover that she was slowly being ground down by the systematic and officially glorified Stalinist paranoia, as if by imperceptible grinding teeth. The traumas of the emotionally isolated dictator had reached far beyond the USSR. His principal goal, to preserve his own power, fell heavily on the most faithful and converted their lives into nightmares of Kafkaesque proportions. Judit took the opportunity, with indirect wording—and always in connection with her own personal problems—to brand the communist leaders "people who compensate for their private misfortunes by attacking each other and who don't hesitate to kill in a spirit of pure persecution frenzy. They have long since forgotten the proletariat, in whose name they claim to act. They always travel first class because they can't stand the smell of the proletariat." But despite this insight, Judit could not forgive Attila for dissociating himself so completely from what he called the "degenerative fascist communists." Their personal and political problems became entangled in an insoluble mess, and at one point Judit tried to kill herself. They later agreed to live apart.

After Attila's death Judit met once, accidentally, with Dr. Rapaport. According to her, the doctor agreed that it had been a mistake to accept Attila for analysis. In one portion of her book, Judit wonders in an insightful and sober way whether Dr. Rapaport really understood at all the intensity of Attila's prolonged suffering. What can the world offer a man whose attachment to his mother forces him to long constantly for a love that can never be returned? The love of a woman is not enough. Nor does a prominent position in society compensate. During his lifetime Attila had received love from an entire nation, especially from the poor. They came flocking wherever he appeared. Judit tells of a teenage worker, earning twelve pengö a week doing hard labor, who always gave seven pengö to his family and had to save the remaining five for transportation, clothing, and food. Once, when he happened to find one pengö that someone had forgotten on a table, he gave it to Attila rather than putting it into his own pocket.

The poor man's coin was more valuable than the rich man's gold. According to Judit, Attila's successes among the wealthy came as a severe shock to him. The lavish dinners at the home of his patron Baron Hatvany caused Attila a great deal of anguish, despite the fact that he was being introduced as the guest of honor, the master of the language, the wonder child. Champagne, imported whiskey, and cognac were suddenly flowing all around him. His stomach, half or completely empty for all his years, was now experiencing caviar and salmon; the cheapest kind of workers' cigarettes were being replaced by the best imported brands. Everything was being offered to him as if he were a feudal lord, with bowing and other expressions of submission worthy of an important and powerful gentleman.

Attila used to end these evenings with a long, solitary walk home, both his stomach and his soul turned upside down. He felt defeated and destroyed. He was out of work, and he didn't belong to any society or any political party. He belonged only to an analyst. When he arrived home, he would inevitably rouse the sleeping Judit, cry, and become aggressive. They would quarrel, and finally Judit would have to put him to bed as if he were an abused child. Once, when he was finally in bed, sobbing, he said suddenly, "Read the poem in my pocket." It was the newly written and now immortal poem, "Mother."

For a week now, again and again,
Thoughts of my mother have racked my brain.
Gripping a basket of washing fast,
On, and up to the attic she passed.

And I was frank and released my feeling
In stamps and yells to bring down the ceiling.
Let someone else have the bulging jackets,
Let her take me with her up to the attic.

She just, giving me no look or thrashing,
Went on, and in silence spread out the washing,
And the kneaded clothes, rustling brightly,
Were twisted and billowing up lightly.
I should not have cried but it's too late for this.
Now I can see what a giant she is.
Across the sky her grey hair flickers through;
In the sky's waters she is dissolving blue.[24]

But his dead mother also became the object of constant re-
proaches. He wrote the poem "Cry Late" in 1935.

I burn with a fever of 98 point 6, and still you do not come.
In a loose girdle of virtue you are stretched beside your lover.
I try to piece you together
from autumn scenes and many dear women,
but I fail, for the fire
burns me to ashes.[25]

The third woman, Márta Vágó, has written the most informative
book about Attila.[26] She was the daughter of a prosperous Jewish
family. The father was a prominent economist, very much at home
in the most influential circles despite his origins. He was a great
lover of literature, music, and the arts, like many Hungarian Jews
of his generation. Márta and Attila met at one of the many parties
that her parents gave at their home, through which the writers,
poets, journalists, and literary critics of the day passed in a
constant stream. Attila was then twenty-three years old, Márta
twenty-five. After an awkward and timid start, an intensely emotional relationship developed between the two, as reflected in
Attila's poems from 1928 and in his many love letters to her, some
of which are published in her book.

Attila appeared in the Vágó family circles like a rare kind of bird,
but he was nevertheless received with warmth and appreciation.
He went along on many outings with the rest of the family and
their friends. Márta's book reveals that she was intensely in love
with Attila. During their frequent long walks through the many
beautiful parts of Budapest, she became entranced by his brilliant
associations, his deep seriousness, and his genius with language.
Nevertheless, Attila failed to transform their relationship into a
sexual one, despite many cunning tries. In the final analysis, her

parents were "always more firm than he was," Márta writes. She once told him in a letter that "I don't know at all if we would be suitable for each other as man and wife, and I would certainly die from an extramarital affair."

Like Koestler, Márta was often amazed by the many contrasting aspects of Attila's personality—his "strange mixture of courage and weakness, his almost infantile sincerity, his total willingness to give himself without hesitation, and kind of male assertiveness revealed by oft-repeated comments that there was nothing that he needed to keep secret. He claimed that everything was permitted to him, he accepted himself as he was and he wanted others to accept him in the same way."

Márta's parents apparently liked Attila at first, as they disregarded the advice of their friends not to let their daughter associate with a proletarian like Attila with such a questionable background.The expressions that Márta cites, and rejects, in describing the reactions of these people were typical of the contempt that members of the upper-middle class of the time had for those in society worse off than they. One expression describes a "person who has fallen from a tree," and another alludes to someone "who cannot quite fill his stomach." The overt class-oriented ruthlessness was one of the facts of life in the semi-feudal Hungarian state.

Attila was acutely aware of his social inferiority. He was hypersensitive and burdened with complexes, but nevertheless was fairly happy in the presence of Márta's family. He often discussed literature with her father, and Attila's contact with the family's literary friends undoubtedly contributed to his maturation as a writer. Some of his famous word contrasts were created during this period. In this circle people lived life as poetry—poetry itself was enormously important to them, even more important than life. Attila's mood varied from exultation, playfulness, and elan to recurring periods of melancholy punctuated by astounding attacks of precipitous honesty about subjects quite personal to him. Márta wrote that Attila was "open and forthright with everyone, without a thought of what might follow. He also could not or would not conceal anything or protect himself from truth. He would talk of his most intimate feelings and seemed free of any social constraints, taking seriously any questions asked of him, even when he was joking. He wanted all his poetry to be understandable and accessible to everyone."

There was virtually no one in the Vágó circle of friends who didn't come under Attila's spell at one time or another, especially as they listened to him recite his poems. It was unanimously agreed that he did that better than even the professionals. Márta writes, "He read for us through the entire evening. He loved to recite poetry, but not only his own works. Never have I heard anyone read poetry so simply, so artistically or with such understanding. When he came upon a particularly good line, he laughed aloud triumphantly, became quite tender and seemed moved, and then he repeated certain words for emphasis. When he read the works of other poets, he breathed in synchrony with the author's breaths and showed delight in the felicitous results and in unexpected masterful expressions of his fellow poets. Again and again, he elicited attention with an outstretched arm, with a pointed finger. He enjoyed his performance so much that he broke into a sweat, glowing with delight and concentrating fully on the outlet of his talent. By modulating his voice and with the full use of his entire body and his soul, he interpreted even the smallest details in the verses of Kosztolányi or other poets dynamically and with intellectual clarity. I have always thought that there is no one as much in love with eternal values as Attila. That is exactly what we learned in our religion classes in school; love with all your heart, all your soul and all your ability."

But the family's friends were constantly warning that Attila would never be molded into any ordinary middle-class pattern and that he was completely unsuitable for a solid marriage with Márta. That fact was reinforced by Attila's total inability or unwillingness to find "boring but necessary" employment. Because of his unending need for money and his habit of borrowing from practically anyone who happened to be nearby, including family friends, and because of his occasional bursts of interest in other women, Márta accused him in a letter of "lacking character." Shortly thereafter, she came to regret that letter deeply. But at the same time, she appreciated the positive sides of Attila's apparently indolent attitude to life. She describes how Attila realized how different he was from others as early as 1919, during the unsuccessful communist revolution. He was then only fourteen years old. The rioting crowds plundered and looted shops and department stores without mercy. Attila took part in the looting, but he gave all that he took to children who loitered around in the street outside but lacked the courage to join in the rioting. He even gave away all the pairs of boots he had taken, and didn't keep a single pair to replace his own worn-out shoes. He was later to display the same attitude toward his possessions and his income. He shared everything he owned with others and, eventually, with the whole world. He could not keep anything for himself.

In the autumn of 1928, Márta decided to study economics and sociology in London. In addition to her studies at the London School of Economics, Márta was anxious to get to know England. Most of her published letters to Attila were from this period. She forced herself to live in one of the slums (a "settlement"), but after several days she returned to a simple middle-class area. Her letters are filled with yearning, love, compassion, and worry for Attila, whom she constantly urged to find employment and to whom she often sent money taken from her own allowance. She made no secret of the fact that the letters that she received from her parents hinted at their increasing concern over her strong involvement with Attila. And yet, at the same time, they treated Attila like a member of the family. Even the family's literary and professional friends wrote to Márta, warning her of Attila's unreliability and irresponsibility. Some who traveled to London went so far as to question Attila's intelligence or to divulge that they had seen Attila with other women.

Attila's letters from this same period give hints of the same desperate longing for a mother figure that he had shown in his relationships with other women. But in the case of Márta, there was also strong evidence for his need for an intellectual playmate. He is aware, however, of the great differences in their attitudes toward practical life. In a letter to Márta written in October 1928, Attila praises her ability to cope with the duties of everyday life. "You are a girl, I am a boy. But yet it is you who can deal with all the necessary chores—they don't seem to cause you very much strain. I become completely unwound, not from work but from the urge to work. You are the fin of the fish but you are also the harpoon thrown into it."

The correspondence between the two broke off in the spring of 1929, coincidental with—or possibly because of—Attila's budding relationship with Judit. Attila and Márta did not meet again until November 1936, by which time everything had changed. Márta had gone through a passionate but failed marriage to a German intellectual, and had also had what she called a nervous breakdown. This time they were together until the spring of 1937, the year of Attila's suicide. They separated when Attila fell in love with Flóra, just before his move to the nursing home.

Even though Márta was still deeply in love with the poet, she finally had become convinced that he was seriously disturbed. He lived by no schedule, he kept no appointments, he often arrived suddenly and unannounced and was frequently irritable, aggressive, distracted, and irrational. All this indicated that "he neither could or would give anything of himself to others." He put everything into his poetry, and he thereby gave to all. He was still quite unable to maintain solid relationships with anyone. He had no patience for waiting for mutual feelings to develop spontaneously and naturally in others. If he were asked to explain or defend his behavior, he became angry and withdrew into himself. He wanted everything immediately—a firm foundation for support, unconditional love—to help him cope with his painful life, a life in which he concentrated his rigorous intellectual activity on his poetry, on the sharpening of concepts, on the crystallization of remarkable confluences of ideas, on a constant struggle to find the perfect mode of expression, the perfect melody and rhyme. Gentler feelings only bubbled up within him whenever he suddenly saw an opportunity to find sustenance, to establish a firm footing. But what he saw was often a mirage. Those who tried to find grounds for interacting with him usually encountered only rugged wilderness.

Attila spent all day lying in his dreary, dirty rented room. He saw light only in the cafés where he spent his nights. Márta quotes from his poem "Eszmélet" (Awakening) written during this period. The last verse describes in beautiful metaphorical terms the transformations of day and night in the context of his constant fixation on trains:

My home's across the railroad. Here
I often watch the whisking trains,
how lighted windows disappear
in waving nights upon the plains.
That is the way the light of days
runs into our eternal night—
I lean upon my arms and gaze
and stand in each compartment's light.[27]

In January 1937, Thomas Mann visited Budapest. The literary magazine *Szép Szó,* to which Attila was a regular contributor, arranged an evening lecture for Mann at the Madach Theater on January 13. Attila was commissioned to write a poem of tribute to Mann. By the afternoon of January 12, Attila had not yet started writing the poem. Márta knew what an honor it was for Attila to have been asked, and she was very concerned. She worried about Attila having a breakdown and about what would happen if the poem was not finished on time. She was irritated by Attila's blasé and self-assured attitude. "Calm down," he said. "I will do it. There is no problem. I can write poems whenever I choose. What I don't know how to do is to live."

Márta thought that this artistic arrogance came from some kind of self-sacrificial attitude. Attila wanted to prove that he could always spit out a poem, whether in response to an inner force or an external request. But she continued to worry, until finally Attila became extremely upset, jumped up, and went out, slamming the door behind him.

One can easily understand Márta's concern. The issue was not only to have the poem finished in time for the lecture, but also to deliver it to the police station for censorship no later than the morning of January 13.

When Márta arrived at the theater the following evening, she learned that Attila had written a wonderful poem, but that the censor had not permitted it to be read to the public. Attila was deathly pale and was trying to telephone the police chief and even the minister of the interior. Márta began to wonder if he was in full possession of his senses. Apparently Attila had written the poem in a café during the night, while his literary friends were making a great deal of noise around him. Attila always looked forward to a large audience and enjoyed reciting his poetry to the

public. As soon as he finished his poem, he showed it to his
friends. They all thought it was a masterpiece. A Hungarian-
speaking German boy in the group at the café immediately
translated it into German, so that it could be presented to Mann.

Welcome to Thomas Mann

Just as the child, by sleep already possessed,
Drops in his quiet bed, eager to rest,
But begs you: "Don't go yet; tell me a story,"
For night this way will come less suddenly,
And his heart throbs with little anxious beats
Nor wholly understands what he entreats,
The story's sake or that yourself be near,
So we ask you: Sit down with us; make clear
What you are used to saying; the known relate,
That you are here among us, and our state
Is yours, and that we are all here with you,
All whose concerns are worthy of man's due.
You know this well: the poet never lies,
The real is not enough; through its disguise
Tell us the truth which fills the mind with light
Because, without each other, all is night.
Through Madame Chauchat's body Hans Castorp sees,
So train us to be our own witnesses.
Gentle your voice, no discord in that tongue;
Then tell us what is noble, what is wrong,
Lifting our hearts from mourning to desire,
We have buried Kosztolanyi; cureless, dire,
The cancer on his mouth grows bitterly,
But growths more monstrous gnaw humanity.
Appalled we ask: More than what went before,
What horror has the future yet in store?
What ravening thoughts will seize us for their prey?
What poison, brewing now, eats us away?
And, if your lecture can cut off that doom,
How long may you still count upon a room?
O, do not speak, and we can take heart then.
Being men by birthright, we must remain men,
And women, women, cherished for that reason.
All of us human, though such numbers lessen.
Sit down, please. Let your stirring tale be said.
We are listening to you, glad, like one in bed,
To see to-day, before that sudden night,
A European mid people barbarous, white.[28]

In 1937, there were few among the Hungarian intelligentsia
who were as able as Attila to foresee the impending threat to
Europe, to humanity, and to human dignity. It was a time for the
Epigonis, for euphemisms, for bourgeois sentimentality in art
and literature. But Attila's voice rang out like a warning bell.

Márta noticed that Mann read the poem with a distressed
expression on his face as he leaned against the wall shortly before
his lecture. He liked it very much, but he had noticed the
commotion that ensued when Attila had tried, to everyone's
consternation, to phone the minister of the interior. Mann went
to Márta, whom he had met earlier together with Attila, and Márta
describes the following short conversation as follows: "He belongs
to you," he said with a quick gesture and a faint smile, "and you
must take care of him. But you must not marry him. I think he
is a manic-depressive or something even worse. Hatvany[29] thinks
that he is just a little *meschugge*," he said, smiling, "but I am afraid
that it is much more serious. He absolutely must get some medical
attention," he added gravely.

"He is already in psychoanalysis," Márta answered.

"Do you really believe in that?"

Márta said yes, with conviction.

Mann asked if she was also in psychoanalysis, and Márta nod-
ded, all the while looking at Mann searchingly. He threw his arms
out like a skeptical but resigned scientist, and said, "Perhaps it will
help. But I hardly think so. But his poem is certainly wonderful
(*wunderschon*)."

One month later, the poem was published in *Szép Szó*. By that
time there was a different censor handling the literary magazines,
and he let it pass. To Márta it was by then quite clear that Attila
was in the process of psychological dissolution. But since she
thought there was a causal connection between Attila's earlier
life, especially his childhood, and his symptoms, she still refused
to believe that the problem represented a mental illness. She
found nothing out of the ordinary in his constant crises, although
she was deeply hurt by his sudden eruptions of violent temper.
In the spring of 1937, when Attila's attentions had turned to Flóra,
his attitude toward Márta swung from one of great affection to
one of repugnant aggressiveness. Their relationship then ended
for the second time. After Attila's admission to the nursing home,

Márta wanted to visit him, but the psychiatrists did not allow her to come.

Márta received news of Attila's death in the form of a telephone invitation to the funeral. That was the hardest blow she had ever experienced, and she never fully recovered from it.

Epilogue

On October 8, 1928, Márta was sitting in her rented room in the slums of London. She could not sleep. The nights were the most difficult in those dirty quarters, where windows could not be opened without soot being blown in and covering everything. When dawn came she was overcome with anxiety, with a longing to be freed from her self-imposed exile, burdened with the demands of her feelings of duty mixed with her trivial everyday problems. She was also worried about the uncertain future of the twenty-three-year-old Attila, about his inability to find a stable job. Along with the complicated family relationships on both sides, these thoughts chased each other around in a vicious self-reinforcing circle. Suddenly she remembered Attila's poem "Place Your Hand on My Forehead, As If Your Hand Were My Hand." Her mood brightened, all her gloomy thoughts vanished. Attila had written the twelve very short lines earlier that same year and had given them to her during their second meeting. The poem is as light as air, clear as crystal, perfect in form and content. It is one of the classics of Hungarian literature, similar to Goethe's "Über allen Gipfeln" in German poetry. It ends with the words, "Watch over me as if others wanted to murder me, as if my life were yours. Love me as if it would be good, as if my heart were your heart."

Márta had earlier described how the shy and embarrassed young man had read the poem to her from a scrap of paper cluttered with pencil marks. Márta, who was probably the first person ever to hear the poem, was completely bewitched. The absolute perfection of the poem reminded her of Mozart's music. It wasn't until much later that she learned that it had been written for her between their first and second meetings.

You do not have to be a young woman or Attila's contemporary to be overwhelmed and "helped" by Attila's writings (see the

chapter entitled "Orpheus"). When I read about Márta's experience in her dreary room in London's slums, I suddenly recalled
a late summer night in August 1944, when I was on my way home
in Budapest. It was the most fateful year for Hungary's Jews, when
eight of every ten of us were killed in the Auschwitz gas chambers,
in military slave camps, or on the long death marches when there
was not enough transportation available. I knew about all this
from the report on Auschwitz that I had read as early as May of
the same year. By August, virtually all my father's family, including
my beloved grandmother, had already been murdered at Auschwitz.
I didn't know how long I would survive, but I didn't think that
it could be for more than a few weeks or months. At the same time,
I was deeply in love for the first time. I had just escorted my
girlfriend home after a long walk through the dark streets on that
summer night. Those of us with Jewish stars sewn onto our
clothing were not allowed to use the trams in the evening. But I
felt wonderful. On my way home, I was completely filled with the
happiness of love, but at the same time I was also fully aware of
our situation. There had just been a lull in the deportations, a
pause that seemed to me only a temporary calm in the storm. The
Jews of the countryside had already been annihilated or were on
their way to an agonizing death. Only we, the Jews of Budapest,
were left—thanks to the intervention of the head of state, Admiral
Horthy, in response to requests from the Pope and the Swedish
king, a reprimanding speech by President Roosevelt, the extensive bombings of Budapest, and perhaps above all, because Mrs.
Horthy had read the smuggled report about Auschwitz. But I
knew that the Germans could decide to depose Horthy any day
and install an extremist Nazi group such as the Arrow Cross party,
to allow the murder of the Jews to resume. This in fact took place
later, on October 15. But my happiness of the moment surpassed
my deeper feelings of anxiety. I realized how absurd this was, but
I searched in vain for words that could express what I felt.
Suddenly I was struck by a few lines from a poem that rose up from
my subconscious. They were the introductory verses from Attila's
late poem "My Native Land." The lines and their full content are
virtually impossible to translate. Just how impossible it was dawned
on me when I tried to produce a verbatim translation. The first
line, "Tonight as I was walking home," is simple. The next line

starts with the words, "I felt. . . ," expressing so precisely my feelings at the time that I can feel the same thing now. But I cannot convey at all the following three words. The poet felt a vibration in the air, but he describes it with an expression that implies a continuous caress. The poet uses a rare verb to describe this movement, a verb that refers to the swinging of a pendulum, back and forth, softly and slowly. It touched the skin like velvet. All of this was expressed by only three unusual words, which would never be combined in ordinary spoken language. Nor would they be brought together in that way by any other poet. Still, with an almost mathematical precision they expressed the feeling that went through me, from head to toe.

The following two lines consist of only five words. The poet writes of jasmines. In her memoirs, Márta writes that Attila wanted to dedicate this poem to her, a work written during the last year of his life, by which time he was in very bad condition. But to Attila's great sorrow, she rejected his offer. When he first read the poem to her, he mentioned that his first impulse was to let the jasmines "spread their aroma." But he suddenly changed his mind and used an amazing word, now inscribed forever, that implies that the jasmines "applauded." It is an image that makes most people lift their heads and listen. According to Márta, the connection between these images came to Attila when he once looked at a jasmine blossom in a light wind. The petals quivered and touched each other. All these images with one word. With three more words, the poet describes the movement of the petals—the soft warmth stirred now and then by a breath of wind on the border between feeling and reality.

The fourth line can readily be translated as "my soul was a dreamy jungle." The remainder of the poem is as overwhelming to the reader as a Bach fugue, building from a quiet thematic introduction to a woven fabric of voices that retain their independent contrapuntal existences. It is a blending that strikes the reader like a mighty, shimmering dome. One can only stand motionless underneath it, amazed, overwhelmed, elevated, ecstatic. This is exactly what I felt on my way home. On his walk home, the poet saw the homeless sleeping in the streets. He was seized by a feeling of unity with them, with the misery of the nation. The diseases and curses of the people parade in front of him: infant mortality, the plight of orphans, premature aging, mental illness, criminality, suicide, indolence, and a thousand other problems awaiting solution. Those in power sit entranced by their own exercise of power, indifferent to the devastation of the people. The poem continues with a crushing attack on the whole feudal system—the landowners, the police, the rigged elections, the bowed backs of the workers, the distrust of the rich by the poor and vice versa, the wary fear that drives everything and everyone, the illusory hope. The son of the people emerges from his past millennium with a small bundle on his back, searching for a caretaker's job instead of destroying his father's grave as he ought to. "But yet, now that I have been exiled to these lands, open yourself to me, my country—I want to be your faithful son. He who wishes to be led on a leash like a circus bear can continue trampling onward, but I will not. I am a poet. Tell your prosecutor that he must not pluck my feathers. You have driven our peasants to the seas. It is now time to give humanity back to humans, to make the Hungarian into a Magyar so that we do not become a German colony."

German colony, I thought in 1944, sitting between the jaws of death. Attila, the prophetic poet then already dead for seven years, saw what was to come long before anyone else. The dreamy jungle of his soul spoke to me as I was on my way home, filled with the happiness of love and the bottomless despair of today and tomorrow. His hopeful spirit spoke to me, I who lacked all illusions. The desperate poet, in the process of losing his final grip, was crying out his encouragement to me, who had already lost my grip but nevertheless was going to survive and attain the freedom that the poet had sought in vain. The dead poet, helpless as a small child, sustained the survivors and will continue to sustain them for many generations to come—regardless of age, social climate, or political system—through the paradoxes of human existence. This is how I remember Attila, as he goes over the horizon to stay forever with us who understand his words.

Part Three

4

Orpheus

Never have we heard aforetime
heard before such charming music,
in the course of all our lifetime,
when the brilliant moon was shining.[1]

A friend who knows me quite well has sent me a short story by C.
J. Burckhart, accompanied by a laconic note saying that it might
interest me.[2] The title in English is, "A Morning at the Bookstore."
What could that possibly mean? My friend knows that he can
count on my curiosity. I put it on my desk, on top of the pile
labeled "general interest." I sometimes allow myself the pleasure,
with some feelings of guilt, of reading material from this pile—
standing, holding a piece of cheese in my left hand and an apple
in the right, the door to the room firmly closed. Who would want
to catch their professor in such an uncivilized pose? I personally
cannot imagine how anyone can sit down at a table to a big lunch
together with friends, talking about the same mundane matters
day after day, while the collective wisdom and experience of all
humanity and the works of the great masters sit there around us,
gathering dust.

 The story starts routinely enough. Do I really want to read this?
Burckhart writes about a visit to a barbershop, where he asks to
have his hair washed. He begins describing in great detail the
unpleasant feeling of having his head lowered into the washbasin
and of the water, the shampooing, the bubbles, and various kinds
of massage. No—I can't read this. How could anyone send this
stuff to me? But while Burckhart remains in this blinded state, his
head covered with soap, he suddenly hears a commotion quite

nearby. A woman employee is arguing loudly with a customer, and calls for the manager. He arrives at the scene and raises his voice even louder than hers—a duet of irritation is raised to the level of a trio. The unthinkable has apparently occurred. A customer has been given the most attentive service possible, with the most expensive lotion, but he cannot pay. In a small, squeaky voice he tries, to no avail, to convince them that he has merely forgotten his wallet and can return immediately with the money. Anyone can say that! We don't even know the gentleman! Nothing like this has ever happened here before! We are a first-class establishment! The voices become more and more irate, and the manager threatens to call the police. And then suddenly Burckhart hears the shaky tenor voice say in a tone of resignation, "You can call and inquire. I am the poet Rainer Maria Rilke." Bang!

With the manager and the employee screaming, "Anyone can say that!" Burckhart gets out of his chair, pushes his protesting barber aside and, with soap still foaming in his hair, walks over to the scene of the melee and announces that he will pay for Rilke.

It is here that the story really begins, but for me it is already over—I have gotten my jolt. I recognize the kind of "electric shock" that the Israeli author Amos Oz talks about in his lectures on literature, the overpowering feeling that comes quite unexpectedly when one is reading the great writers. My own literature-loving gang in Budapest used to talk about the "spine syndrome," a shiver that suddenly races from the neck to the small of the back, a radical change in the state of consciousness, if ever so fleeting.

But I certainly have not just finished reading something great—only an absurd everyday event of the most banal sort. Well, that is exactly what it is all about. How could such an ordinary human being who has carelessly misplaced his wallet, and who finds himself in such a meaningless situation in that ordinary barbershop, utter this phrase in such an offhand way? How could a person ask for a shampoo and order the most expensive kind of hair lotion, insisting all the while that he is the great poet, the author of these lines:

Du bist die Zukunft, grosses Morgenrot
über den Ebenen der Ewigkeit
Du bist der Hahnschrei nach der Nacht aer Zeit

der Tau, die Morgenmette und die Maid
der fremde Mann, die Mutter und der Tod.

You are the future, the great sunrise red
above the broad plains of eternity.
You are the cock-crow when time's night has fled,
You are the dew, the matins, and the maid,
the stranger and the mother, you are death.[3]

These lines follow and console me, lead me through life and arise when all seems dark and unendurable—with the timeless-ness, the great promise of freedom, the intoxication that permits me to continue, slowly and patiently, toward the night.

Was he then just an ordinary human being, like you and me? Has he stood in line, has he gone to the toilet? Could he say simply, "I am the poet," rather than "The Poet," just as one might say, "I am the doctor/the mailman/the tax assessor"? How could he bring himself to utter that name, those three words, those seven syllables that should only be printed with eternal, unalter-able letters?

Where is this feeling leading me?

Orpheus—one of Rilke's most beloved figures, the stone relief that leads directly to "the souls' wondrous mine" (*der Seelen wunderliches Bergwerk*). It's an archetypal symbol for all poets:

Er ist einer der bleibenden Boten,
der noch weit in die Türen der Toten
Schalen mit rühmlichen Früchten hält.

For he is a herald who is with us always,
holding far into the doors of the dead
a bowl with ripe fruit worthy of praise.[4]

It is exactly there that we can most easily find him, at the gates of hell, at the entrance to the land of death. The great Hungarian poet Attila József (see the chapter entitled "Attila József") has expressed this in four limpid lines that resemble a children's song (and can therefore be perceived even by those who do not understand Hungarian) that introduce a collection of his poems. It is as light as a feather, yet full of meaning:

Aki dudás akar lenni
pokolra kell annak menni

ott kell annak megtanulni
hogyan kell a dudát fujni.

He who wants to play the bagpipe
must first descend to hell. Only there
can he learn how to blow the bagpipe.

In classical mythology and in many theatrical and musical versions, Orpheus seeks admission to hell but is met by the Furies, who threaten to tear him into thousands of pieces. They want him first to be seized with fear and despair:

The angry Furies will fill him with terror
Cerberus' howl will frighten him if he is not a god.[5]

Orpheus begs for mercy, but in vain. "Furies, monsters, angry phantoms. Have mercy on my tormenting pain!" But in response he hears only implacable and repeated "No," hitting him like hammer blows. He reaches for his harp and sings, "A thousand torments have I also (*anch'io*) suffered, just like you, forlorn shadows. I carry my own Hell within me."

The Furies notice with astonishment that their anger is beginning to abate. "What mild, strange feeling is softly soothing our implacable fury?"

Orpheus continues his singing:

Men tiranne voi sareste
al mio pianto, al mio lamento
se provaste un sol momento,
cosa sia languir d'amor.

You would be less cruel towards
my cry and my sorrow if you could feel,
at least for a moment, the languish of love.

Now the Furies can resist no longer. They relent, bow down in front of the singer, and lie sprawled on the ground. Finally they arise to celebrate his triumph: "Open the gates for the trumphant (*al vincitor*), he should be free to go where he wants!"

Can iron gates be opened, can the hatred of hell be softened with song? What are all the Furies of hell compared with the extermination camps of the Nazis? The monumental film "Shoah" by Claude Lanzmann begins with an idyllic boat ride near the site of the first annihilation camp in Chelmno, Poland. It was here that the first mass murders took place on December 7, 1941, using exhaust from trucks to gas people. The corpses were burned openly each day, and a total of 400,000 people died there.

Simon Srebnik, a somewhat obese, mild-mannered, middle-aged man is seen walking around with Lanzmann on the green, flowering meadow at the edge of the woods. Where were the fires? Just over here. They then continue their ride down that same peaceful river on which Srebnik traveled as a young teenager, guarded by the SS. The guards and the Polish farmers listened as Srebnik sang, and to this day they can remember the song: "A small white house is forever in my memory, I dream about it every night." The SS men wanted to hear that sentimental song over and over, and the boy sang and survived. He was the only survivor among the hundreds of thousands. "When the soldiers go by, all the girls open their doors and windows." In Lanzmann's film he sings the song again with a strange, distant look in his eyes. The Polish farmers listen and some of the older ones recognize his voice. They seem unconcerned about those who were gassed or burned to death, but they seem quite happy that the young boy, now no longer so young, has survived and that they can hear his voice once again.

Songs that can move mountains. The Orpheus legend, one of mankind's most irresistible archetypes. I know of only one surviving epos that has used a singer-poet as its central figure, the Finnish epos *Kalevala.* The old but steadfast Väinämöinen, the son of the sea maiden Ilmatar, was born when he was already six hundred years old, just as the earth, sun, moon, and stars were created. He was often called "born with the sun" or the "primeval magician." He was able to subjugate all with his song, as illustrated by the contest of wisdom and singing with the young hero Joukahajnen. Joukahajnen had berated Väinämöinen when the latter refused to meet him in combat, but he had no way of predicting what was to happen when Väinämöinen began to sing:

Lakes swelled up, and earth was shaken,
And the coppery mountains trembled,
And the mighty rocks resounded.
And the mountains clove asunder;
On the shore the stones were shivered. [6]

The young hero Joukahajnen doesn't have a chance. He sinks waist deep into the swamp, his sword and shield are crushed, and he can free himself only by promising his sister Aino in marriage to Väinämöinen. He returns to his home, feeling ashamed and guilty for having sold his sister, but he finds to his great surprise that

joyous clapped her hands his mother,
both her hands she rubbed together.[7]

She can imagine no greater honor than to have Väinämöinen as a son-in-law. However, the planned marriage ends in tragedy, for Aino chooses death over marriage to an old man.

But Väinämöinen's power is undiminished. Does his magic merely reflect old superstitions? That is what one might believe until one reads what happened when he made a new harp (*kantele*). Väinämöinen first offers to allow others to play upon it, but all does not go well:

Played the young and played the aged,
Likewise played the middle-aged,
Played the young and moved their fingers,
Tried the old, whose heads were shaking,
But they drew no music from it,
Nor composed a tune when playing.[8]

They are about to throw away the stringed instrument because they cannot stand its terrible noise, but

With its tongue the harp made answer,
As the *kantele* resounded
"No, I will not sink in water
Nor will rest beneath the billows,
But will play for a musician,
Play for him who toiled to make me."[9]

And then it happens:

Väinämöinen, old and steadfast,
He the great primeval minstrel
Presently stretched out his fingers,
Washed his thumbs, the harp for playing.
And his hands he placed beneath it,
Then he spoke the words which follow,
"Come ye now to listen to me,
Ye before who never heard me,
Hear with joy my songs primeval
While the *kantele* is sounding."[10]

All creatures—humans, the animals of the forest, fish, birds, even the angels in heaven—listen as Väinämöinen sings. Even the sun, the moon, and the fire come to listen. The result is tragedy, because the sun and moon are abducted. But before that happens, another far more important event occurs that reveals the Orpheus-like power of Väinämöinen:

Then the aged Väinämöinen,
Played one day, and played a second,
There was none among the heroes,
None among the men so mighty,
None among the men or women,
None of those whose hair is plaited,
Whom he did not move to weeping,
And whose hearts remained unmelted.
Wept the young and wept the aged,
All the married men were weeping,
Likewise all the married women,
And the half-grown boys were weeping,
All the boys, and all the maidens,
Likewise all the little children,
When they heard the tones so wondrous,
And the noble sage's music.[11]

A great opera singer once said in an interview, "Do not tell me that I sing beautifully. That doesn't mean anything. But tell me when my singing had moved you. That's important to know."

Song, yes. Music, the wordless language of emotions. But how can words, the increasingly weakened and bereft instrument of rational communication, acquire such power in the hands of a poet? How can Orpheus move us so deeply without singing, just through the use of words?

In a letter dated August 26, 1853, Gustave Flaubert writes, "What seems to me the highest and the most difficult in Art is not that it manages to make us laugh or cry, to relieve our desires or angers, but that it can act as Nature itself and make us dream. Truly great works of art do that. They have a calm exterior and their effect is incomprehensible. However, Rabelais, Michelangelo, Shakespeare, Goethe are unrelenting, their works are without end, infinite and vast in their scope. Through small gaps we can see deep chasms. Below, all is darkness, one is overcome by dizziness. But a curious calm hovers over all."

Chasms, darkness, dizziness, dreams, nightmares.

In one of his most impenetrable but powerfully suggestive poems, Edgar Allan Poe finds himself in a land of memory.[12] It is a deserted landscape in which the sky is ashen gray, the leaves withered, dried, and brittle.

The eerie haunted landscape is "by the dim lake of Auber, in the misty mid region of Weir"—imaginary names whose sound intensifies the atmosphere of loneliness and abandonment. It is reminiscent of how Dante went astray in the dark forest without even knowing why he happened to be there.

The poet remembers that he has been there before, together with "Psyche my soul." Here the reader, or at least I, suddenly have an insight into one of the bottomless chasms described by Flaubert. The stroll into the past with Psyche leads to catastrophe, and afterward, Psyche is gone.

The poet recalls the fateful walk:

Here, once, through an alley Titanic,
Of cypress, I roamed with my Soul—
Of cypress, with Psyche my Soul.

During these days, the poet's heart was "volcanic," it erupted rivers of lava,

As the scoriac rivers that roll
As the lavas that restlessly roll
Their sulphurous currents down Yaanek
In the ultimate climes of the Pole—

That groan as they roll down Mount Yaanek,
In the realms of the boreal Pole.

   Literary critics and psychologists have often interpreted these
words as sexual symbols, the ejaculate on its way toward the pole
of the female body. But do we really have to limit our imagination
to something quite so specific and narrow? Is it not more likely
that the inner volcano and its restless rivers of lava reflect the past
and forebode the future?

   The poet and his soul walked unsuspectingly through the
deserted landscape. But suddenly,

. . . as the night was senescent
And star-dials pointed to morn—
As the star dials hinted of morn—

the poet saw a strange light at the end of the alley:

At the end of our path a liquescent
And nebulous lustre was born,
Out of which a miraculous crescent
Arose with a duplicate horn—
Astarte's bediamonded crescent
Distinct with its duplicate horn.

   The poet is seized by a feeling of euphoria. It must have been
a good omen, a sign of mercy from a higher being.
   But Psyche doesn't trust the star and has no faith in "her pallor."

Oh, hasten,!—oh, let us not linger!
Oh, fly!—let us fly!—for we must.
In terror she spoke; letting sink her
Wings until they trailed in the dust—
In agony sobbed, letting sink her
Plumes till they trailed in the dust—
till they sorrowfully trailed in the dust.

   But the poet could see only hope, and was convinced that the
light would

. . .lead us aright—
We safely may trust to a gleaming

That cannot but guide us aright
Since it flickers up to Heaven through the night.

He pacified Psyche, kissed her, and "tempted her out of her gloom." They continued walking toward "the end of the vista," but suddenly were stopped by the door to a tomb.

And I said:—"What is written, sweet sister,
On the door of this legended tomb?"
She replied—"Ulalume—Ulalume!—
'Tis the vault of thy lost Ulalume."

This was an unrelenting shock, the gray ashes and withered leaves of depression:

Then my heart it grew ashen and sober
As the leaves that were crisped and sere.

He was overcome by the memory of that day in October when he journeyed there with his dead beloved.

All roads were barred. The poet is alone in that "ghoul-haunted woodland." Psyche is no longer there, the road leads nowhere, the depression can no longer be lifted. This is the eternal, the only theme for Poe's writing. It has reached its ultimate perfection in "The Raven," a poem that has influenced many generations of readers in many lands.

In the foreword to a new edition of selected works by Poe,[13] W. H. Auden divides Poe's poems into two classes. Some could have been written by any of a number of other poets of the same period. Others could only have been written by Poe. "Ulalume" is cited as the foremost example of the latter category. "The Raven" is so obvious that there is no need even to mention it.

"The Raven" has inspired some of the greatest poets of all Western and some other languages to render this untranslatable poem in their own language. It was first translated into French by no less a poet than Charles Baudelaire. He was probably the greatest among the French lyrical travelers through hell, the prototype for "le poète maudit," the damned poet. Baudelaire's own poetry was strongly influenced by Poe. He called "The Raven" translation his greatest challenge.

Poe himself insisted, however, that "The Raven" was written without emotion, with pure cold calculation. In his essay, "The Philosophy of Composition," first published in George Rex Graham's *The Gentleman's Magazine* in 1846, Poe describes the origins of "The Raven." The goal of the poem was to make the greatest possible impression. Just how can that be done? First and foremost, the reader's interest must be awakened. One must express oneself as originally as possible, because that is most likely to entice the reader to listen to what is being said. But what kinds of effects should one aim for among all those that emotions, the intellect, and the soul are susceptible to? Poe expresses his amazement that no previous writers have described in detail the route toward a perfect composition. He suspects that this might be due to the vanity of writers, their wish to preserve the illusion of poetic ecstasy or even their reluctance to permit the public a peek behind the scenes of writing.

Should we believe him, or should we instead side with Baudelaire, who claims in *La genèse d'un poëme* that Poe's essay on the "The Raven" has its origins in a perverse kind of ambition? Did he pretend to be so much less inspired than he truly was out of a curious sense of vanity? Could he have tried to belittle the obvious role of his keen talent by pretending that his composition was essentially an act of will? Baudelaire believes that this is precisely the case, but at the same time he points to Poe's great passion for logical analysis, his oft-stated demand that a writer must be fully aware of the very last line of his work even when he is writing the first line.

In his own view, how did Poe come to write "The Raven"?

The first step was to determine the length of the poem. It must be short enough to be read in one sitting. Otherwise, the trivial events of everyday life would threaten to interrupt and destroy the overall impression of continuity so important for a piece of art to convey its message. In prose this limitation can be averted, but never in poetry. On the other hand, a piece of poetic writing should also not be too short. A poem must cause the reader to feel an intense effect for a continuous period of time.

How long, then, should a poem ideally be? Poe decided that the poem should be one hundred lines long. In actuality, "The Raven" consists of one hundred and eight lines.

What effect should be made on the reader? How can a poem be crafted to effect most or—ideally of course—all readers? What is it in a poem that most readers need to experience that feeling of sublime pleasure? "The contemplation of the beautiful." By "beauty," Poe does not refer to any specific characteristic of the poetic object itself. He speaks rather of an intense effect on the reader, an uplifting of the soul, something much more than an effect on the intellect or emotions. But then who or what is the soul; of what is it made beyond feelings and intellect? Is Poe referring to the same Psyche who becomes his companion during his fateful walk through the Weir woods, along the misty Lake Auber, before the Raven has irrevocably cast its shadow over him? Is the poet still able to give us the most intense pleasure through his poetry even though his own soul is already lost? Yes, that is exactly what he succeeds in doing. But in his essay, Poe speaks to us with a different voice, the cool and critical literary voice, hidden behind a protective facade, a mask of logic. He continues:

Without question, the exaltation of the soul can be achieved most easily through poetry, the special province of the soul itself. Prose provides an intellectually more satisfying avenue toward an analysis of truth, toward an emotional experience and an emotional catharsis. Prose demands precision, but feelings demand empathy. The reader who shares the writer's passions is able to understand him immediately. The exaltation of the soul is something entirely different. In truth, it is quite the opposite of those effects that one might achieve through prose. Poetry can certainly convey truth and passion, but that cannot be its principal purpose. It should instead be used for the elevation of the real effect in exactly the same way that a musical dissonance serves to define the final harmonic effect. Poetry must strive for the exaltation that only verse can create.

What tone should be struck to accomplish such an effect? A great poem can move a sensitive reader to tears. That capacity to move readers depends above all on conveying feelings of sorrow, loss, and sadness. Melancholy is the most appropriate of all poetic moods.

After having determined the length, the desired effect, and the mood of a poem, Poe searches for a key word, a kind of fulcrum for the entire structure. This can most easily be achieved through a refrain, but that is accompanied by a certain risk. The refrain might easily become a burden. The pleasure in a repetitive phrase might readily become wearisome. This problem might be solved through the choice of a refrain whose exact wording can be varied but whose sound can be repetitious and uniform. With that, the basic mood is retained, but a new and astonishing effect can be achieved.

What kind of refrain should it be? Of course, it must be short. If it to allow variation, it should not consist of more than a single word. What sort of word should be used at the close of each verse to provide the tone and the sound, to set the mood for the entire poem? The combination of *o* and *r* seems to be the most suitable sound. Poe's choice of the word "nevermore" falls as timely as a ripe apple from a tree. In his search for the ideal refrain, one that can be repeated and varied, that word carried the right musical quality to convey the melancholy mood that Poe wished to create. "It would have been completely impossible to overlook the word *nevermore*. It was the first word to come into my mind."

How right Poe is!

Among the Swedish translators of "The Raven," Victor Rydberg chooses the word *förbi*, meaning past in time, while Leif Furhammar's raven says *allt förgår*, meaning everything vanishes. Those words determines the entire tone of the poem, and the translation by Furhammar seems to catch the mood of the word most faithfully. Among the many Hungarian translators, Dezsö Kosztolányi was the most eminent poet, but his choice of the word *sohasem* (shohashem), although literarily correct, misses most of the mood. Another great poet, Árpád Tóth, used the word *sohamár* (shohamaar), also correct from a literary point of view but somewhat artificial. However, this word does preserve the appropriate atmosphere. The wonderful German translation by U. Stadtmann is faithful to the music and the context of the poem, but loses some of its dark tone through the use of the obvious German word *nimmermehr*. The same occurs with *aldrei meir* in Einar Benediktssonar's Icelandic translation. The Hebrew translation by Zeev Jabotinsky catches more of the original mood through the use of a quite artificial construct consisting of the four words *al ad ein dor*, meaning "there will be no appropriate epoch for that." One of the many Russian translators, Badmónt, chooses the literarily correct word *nekogda*, while Zeev Jabotinsky completely gives up on trying to find a suitable word in his Russian translation, preferring to let the raven utter the original English "nevermore."

For Baudelaire, *nevermore* is a profound and mystical word, as awesome as infinity, a word that has been uttered by countless taut lips since the beginning of time. He also does not even try to find a French word with the same tone, and is content to use the literarily correct *jamais plus*.

How did Poe continue after having come up with the correct refrain? The problem was to find a pretext for the repetitious use of "nevermore." It was difficult to combine the demand for such monotony with our notions of how a rational being uses language. It seemed more logical to use a nonrational animal, but one with at least a limited ability to "speak." A parrot was the first and most obvious choice, but after some further thought, Poe replaced it with a raven, a creature that can also learn a few words but that fits more appropriately into the atmosphere with which Poe was trying to infuse the poem.

After having determined the length, the mood, and the refrain of the poem and having chosen the ominous and foreboding bird—if we are to believe Poe's own account—he next had to chose a subject. What subject is the most melancholy of all, one that everyone can understand? Death and decay. When is death most poetic? When it strikes at beauty. "The death of a beautiful woman is unquestionably the most poetical topic in the world —and equally it is beyond doubt that the lips best suited for such a topic are those of a bereaved lover."

How might these two ideas be combined—the grieving lover and the raven, monotonously repeating "nevermore"? It seemed important to use the same word to convey a number of different meanings. One therefore had to envision a raven answering questions posed by the lover. The first answer was meant to be both humorous and trivial, the second more portentous, and the third threatening. Through his own anguished questions, the original nonchalance of the lover is transformed into a nightmarish atmosphere pervaded by superstition, passion, self-torture, and despair. The event of a raven flying in through an open window, the rhythm, tone, sadness, and increasingly threatening

presence of the big black bird uttering the message that all hope
is gone—all these transform the scene into one of "delicious" but
"most intolerable sorrow."

After having come thus far in his planning of the poem, Poe was
finally prepared to pick up his pen. But in fact he did not start
at the beginning. He first wrote the third verse from the end:

"Prophet," said I, "thing of evil—prophet still if bird or devil!
By that Heaven that bends above us—by that God we both adore—
Tell this soul with sorrow laden, if, within the distant Aidenn,
It shall clasp a sainted maiden whom the angels name Lenore—
Clasp a rare and radiant maiden whom the angels name Lenore."
Quoth the Raven "Nevermore!"

In his further examination—or rather his rationalization—of
the origins of "The Raven," Poe turns in his essay to a very
professional and technical discussion of the rhythm, form, and
alliterations that he chose to combine to create a unique effect.
He then comes to the question of how the mourning lover and
the raven are to meet. It would have been quite natural, but quite
wrong, to have them meet in the woods or in the open fields. But
the choice of a clearly defined, closed room was "absolutely
necessary" to create the appropriate mood—it was like the frame
of a picture. Only in that way could the poem attain the "moral
power" needed to force the reader to concentrate and be en-
grossed. Poe never loses sight of that goal, either in his poetry or
his prose.

Poe describes the lover, sitting in the well-furnished study where
he had so often been with her, but where she was never again to
appear. He describes the stormy night, the hesitant knock on the
window, the bust of Pallas over the doorway, and the deliberate
and planned effect of the raven's fantastic and dramatic entry.
The poem develops simultaneously along realistic and supernatural levels. A realistic background is provided by the flight of the
bird out of the storm and by the student's attempt to escape from
his depression. The words uttered by the student just before the
raven's entry give us immediate insight into Poe's own flight from
the ever-present threat of the depression that would eventually
defeat him:

vainly I had sought to borrow.
From my books surcease of sorrow
sorrow for the lost Lenore.

The student-poet is never to succeed in freeing himself from the
shadow of the raven. The poem ends with the same motif as in
"Ulalume," but expressed in even clearer terms:

and my soul from out that shadow,
that lies floating on the floor
Shall be lifted—nevermore.

Was this poem really written by cold, deliberate calculation
merely to impress the reader?

I continue reading Poe's biography. His father and mother
were famous actors. The father deserted his family shortly after
their second son, Edgar, was born. The mother died when he was
only two years old, and the children were divided between two
different sets of foster parents. It was a stormy childhood. Edgar
had quite a good record in school, but after a short military career
he was court-martialed and discharged for disobeying orders. He
had published poems and novels by the time he was a teenager,
and his work was well received by the critics. He was hired by a
newspaper as a literary critic, but was reprimanded for his drunken
and disorderly behavior. At twenty-seven he married Virginia
Clemm, a fourteen-year-old girl whom he had known since she
was eight. His job at the newspaper was in jeopardy and his
financial situation was equally unstable. He became a freelance
writer but, despite the fact that the he was able to publish many
poems and stories, his financial insecurity forced him to consider
giving up his writing career. Conflicts erupted, friendships dissolved, literary contracts were cancelled. He proceeded to publish horror stories, thrillers, and mysteries, becoming the father
of the detective story. In 1842, Virginia was stricken with tuberculosis, coughing up blood, close to death. Although she recovered, her recuperation was not complete, and Poe's existence
continued to be tenuous. He fought increasingly difficult battles
against his financial problems and his alcoholism. His chances for
permanent employment vanished completely. But his productiv-
ity continually increased, and he published numerous satires,

poems, and reviews. In 1844, Poe moved to New York and became more and more popular. The following year "The Raven" was published in the *New York Mirror*. It was an instant and enormous success with both general readers and critics, and after numerous editions it was imitated by other writers. He was a favorite of the New York literary elite. But Virginia again fell seriously ill and required constant care and treatment. The year 1846 was characterized by illness, depression, and financial difficulties. Although Poe himself was not well, he continued to publish even as he became involved in controversy and in a lawsuit against a literary critic. Ironically, as he fell into an advanced state of disintegration, his writings earned an international reputation and were translated into several foreign languages.

Virginia died in January 1847. Poe became very ill, and after being nursed by friends, he regained strength and produced two additional poems, one of which was "Ulalume." He attributed his previous alcoholism to the constant attention Virginia had required during her illness. He went through several short-lived love affairs, but continued to write. In 1848 and 1849, Poe again became ill; he was confused and suffered from delusions of persecution. He again became engaged. He was found in the street, in a state of delerium tremens, and died in October 1849.

Was it a deliberate, calculating, and self-serving person who wrote "The Raven"? Just another writer who dies of delerium tremens? I don't believe that for a moment!

Of course, Poe wanted to create certain effects. He was a skilled professional, a literary critic and a master of language and its moods. His novels create the same effect as films by Alfred Hitchcock, "the master of suspense." Poe was virtually without peer and earned this title more than a century before Hitchcock. Success in the usual sense could not have been his principal motivation. This is why the American critics could not forgive him. His aversion or inability to use his enormous talent for practical and egoistic purposes must have been perceived as an insult to the American dream. It was no coincidence that no tombstone was placed on Poe's grave for twenty-six years after his death. Was his motive to allay his own suffering, "to borrow surcease of sorrow" by communicating with others who were ready to listen? Is his poem a masterful verbalization of an inner soliloquy whose purpose corresponds to that of his colleague and admirer Baudelaire, as described in the introductory lines "*sois sage, ô ma douleur, et tiens-toi plus tranquille*" (be wise, my pain, and stay quiet)? Are we so deeply moved by his poem because we know that the final shadow is about to envelop us all, even though we cannot speak of it? Is it possible that the response of readers depends on an insight into the poet's battle with anguish and depression—a battle that was transiently successful but one that Poe would eventually lose? Is *anch'io* (I too) the most important word from Orpheus? Does Orpheus's overwhelming strength come from his ability to convey the feeling that his suffering is also yours and mine? Is it because he is able to convey the fact that the collective suffering of our species is, at the same time, the unique pain of every individual? Is it through Orpheus that we dare to experience our basic and eternally tragic human condition?

That might indeed be the case. But our affinity with Orpheus can be muffled and our communication impeded by many kinds of barriers. Some are obvious and trivial—the barriers of language, fear or dislike of the author, his era, his social class, his presumed or actual political affiliation, his cultural legacy and frames of reference, his choice of words, and his style. But the life of the reader is probably more important.

Budapest, 1986

I am visiting the writer György Konrád, the most articulate voice of protest against the communist regime in contemporary Hungarian literature. He is a master of the language, a writer who combines poetic vision with an uncompromising and penetrating analysis of political lies, including those of the liberal communists. It was his work that at an early stage shed light on the ways in which language and concepts have been misused and divested of their meaning, long before others were able to appreciate such problems. It is not entirely without good reason that he was considered "dangerous," even during the relatively liberal regime of Janos Kádár. Several of Konrád's books have been published only in Swedish, whereas others have been translated into a number of languages.

I am talking with one of Konrád's friends, a young physician in his thirties. Although he is in general just as familiar with Hungarian literature as the most knowledgeable young people of my generation were, I am amazed to find out that the greatest poets from the turn of the century and the period between the two world wars—writers like Endre Ady, Mihály Babits, and Dezső Kosztolányi—seem not to be as significant to him as they were to us. Is that really possible?

Ady was one of the greatest figures of modern poetry in Central and Eastern Europe. He was a writer who provided a bridge between Baudelaire and the expressionist and surrealist poets. He captured his readers with equal strength when he expressed individual anxiety or reflected the perilous condition of his homeland on the brink of the First World War, the collapse of the Austro-Hungarian double monarchy, and the imminent revolution and counterrevolution. He was a primal source of power, one who could strike a responsive chord even in my postwar, middle-class, disillusioned generation. He was a unique figure in Hungarian literature, without equal in all of European literature, with the possible exception of Eino Leino, the Finnish poet. Ady was also the uncompromising defender of the most important right of each artist: to be heard before the coming apocalypse. Is it really possible that he is no longer of interest today?

How about Babits, the reserved poet, the classicist, the greatest virtuoso of the Hungarian language, Ady's opposite pole, who spoke so subtly of hidden sorrows during an era when other writers wore their bleeding hearts on their sleeves?

I ask, "How about Kosztolányi?"—the writer of childhood anguish and adult nostalgia, sensitive but never maudlin; lyrical, symbolic, and sharply satirical, master of contrapuntal verse, a great writer who could convey double meanings and subtle innuendos, who could expose human mendacity with an anatomical-like dissection of human interactions; the unifier of post-psychoanalysis, romanticism, and rationalism.

"Yes," the young physician answers. "Everything you say is true. They are, and will remain, great poets. But they don't help me very much."

"Who does sustain you, what helps? What do you mean by 'don't help?' "

"There is only one writer of that era who, to some extent, does help me, and that is Attila József."

How happy I am to hear that! The name itself gives me the same kind of shiver, almost an electric shock, as I get from the name Rilke. Who can possibly ever forget him?

So it is József who helps, but only to some extent? Who is it then who truly helps?

He mentions György Petri, an obscure poet whom I do not know. The following day, I buy a collection of his poetry.

The language is unsophisticated, sparsely worded, harsh, dark. This is not a master, but rather a poet of protest. The state-sanctioned crimes of the Stalin regime and the tragic Hungarian revolt of 1956 stand out as the central unhealed wounds of his work. There is one poem about Imre Nagy, the prime minister from 1955 to 1956 who became the leader of the revolt more through the pressure of events than through his own free will, and who was later executed despite such assurances. In his poem, Petri is demanding the right to talk and write about this awkward, insecure, somewhat downtrodden, and naive man who first tried in vain to lead—or at least to turn back the avalanche—but who then became seduced by the mirage of his nation's euphoria and unrealistic expectations. The poem ends with the terrible awakening on an early morning in November, as the Russians began shooting in Budapest.

I read further. Siege, collapse, and ruin, the vestiges of old cultures like long-forgotten sets in an abandoned theater. Among his favorite themes are recurring quotations from Baudelaire, "*le poète maudit.*" I can sense how the circle is trying unsuccessfully to close. The hell of Petri differs from the hell of Baudelaire and Poe. The difference is hard to define, but is not merely linguistic. The lonely, pessimistic, and sometimes delightedly morbid *détresse* of Baudelaire has little in common with the shattered dreams of the disappointed socialist Petri. Nonetheless, Petri obviously finds kinship and support in Baudelaire as he tries to describe his dark and frigid hopelessness, when he paints his caricatures of the triumphs of evil, stupidity, and falsehood—expressions like "flaming dung-heap of hatred," "piss-drenched trash," and "the mold of madness and collapse."

I understand my highly literate young colleague, but at the same time I do not understand him. Is he and his generation most moved by the increasingly free—but still not completely unthreatened—voice of protest? Is that really the most important form of expression for a poet, or is it only the recent product of the crimes and muzzled speech of the Stalinist and post-Stalinist eras?

Perhaps so, but I do not think that this form of poetry is going to be long lived. Protest writers come and go. Poe, Dante, and Rilke have messages of timeless relevance that live up to the memorable comment from Poe to Baudelaire, first published in *Southern Literary Messenger* in July 1836: "Aristotle, with singular assurance, has declared poetry the most philosophical of all writings."

But will the timeless messages of poetry continue to be heard? Will there be readers left who can still close their eyes, listen, seek out the voice of Orpheus, his *anch'io*, to calm the Furies and open the gates of hell? Or has the abuse of language through politics and advertising irreparably damaged its credibility? Has the increasingly stereotyped and vapid language of television hosts, stewardesses, telephone operators, secretaries, and even those engaged in everyday conversation caused us to forget that words have the ability to move us more powerfully than anything else—yes, even more than music, the most magical of all art forms? Are we headed toward a society like that of Ingmar Bergman's film *Silence*, in which communication is possible only between people who cannot understand each other's language? Is this leading to the logically consistent end portrayed in Bergman's *Persona,* in which speech is nonexistent?

Jerusalem, 1978

There are rumors going around that a new kind of rabbi occasionally visits the City, the holiest city for all rabbis. He is Shlomo Carlebach, an American, and he plays pop music on his guitar and sings about God and Jerusalem, while jumping up and down, I am told, seized with enthusiasm. Can that be possible?

We are all squeezed together in the inner court of a medieval building in the Old City. The place is filled with young people, sitting on chairs or on the ground or peering in on us through fenestrations in the walls. There is an air of expectancy, but no one has yet appeared on the stage. The atmosphere is relaxed, but soon the noise of the crowd increases and the intensity of the original concentration gives way to restlessness and some irritation. After a half hour, some young men wearing *kippahs*, traditional religious skullcaps, appear on stage with their guitars. They begin playing and singing, but no one is listening. The noise of the crowd continues unabated as if nothing has happened.

Finally, after another hour, Carlebach himself appears. He is not a very attractive man—bald, fat, elderly. He begins tuning his guitar as the crowd noise continues. But suddenly he begins, at first quietly but then louder and louder, singing, playing, and whistling, mixing the usual pop style so popular just then with liturgical songs and with nostalgic and lamenting Chassidic tunes, so rich in symbolism. He sings about Shabbat, the bride, the atmosphere of Friday night, and about the dialogue with God. But above all he sings of Jerusalem, the golden city. As he reaches the emotional climax of his song, he jumps several times into the air.

Like a cloudy mixture of incompatible liquids beginning to separate, the noise of the crowd dissipates and is replaced by a deathly silence, a mood of concentration that I have experienced only at concerts by great masters. This man, however, is no great master. He would never survive in the unforgiving competitive world of show business.

I look around and see mostly Americans and young Jews from many other parts of the world—and only a few Israelis. They are listening to their favorite form of music, the kind of music they have sung, and to which they have made love, but which has not been quite enough for them. Why, otherwise, would they have all made their way here, with their backpacks and sleeping bags? Most have arrived by inexpensive student flights and are staying wherever they can in the country. They can be found on the beaches of the Mediterranean Sea, the Red Sea, the Dead Sea, or the Sea of Galilee. But some are attracted more powerfully to Jerusalem, the eternal city of the spirit, and it is here that they suddenly are coming face to face with their own Dionysian ecstasy, a feeling that has to do not so much with eroticism, previously their only goal, but more with the Shabbat, God, and Jerusalem.

Sublimated libido? A yearning for a spiritual life? I do not know, but it is obvious that Carlebach is reaching into their dreams.

Isn't that precisely what poets have always done? Yes, probably so. It is possible that I was a bit narrow-minded in my judgment of my Hungarian colleague. Poets of anguish and depression, who wage a constant struggle against suicide, are able to bring support to like-minded readers. The writer of political protest and the spiritual rabbi can play equally important roles for their different audiences.

But isn't there anyone who can speak to us all?

In one of his incomparable essays, Lewis Thomas wonders what we would do if we were suddenly to come into contact with members of a civilization from outside our solar system. Suppose that we could send them short messages with brief presentations of the most important features of our culture. It would take many hundreds of years before these messages would reach their destination and for the answer to return to us. What would we send?

"It's obvious, of course," Thomas answers. "Johann Sebastian Bach." But then, after a moment of reflection, he adds, "No, that is not possible. It would be bragging."

Part Four

5

The Ultimate Fear of the Traveler Returning from Hell

Was Dante in hell? Did Strindberg experience inferno? Yes, in a way, but they managed to escape and write about it for our delight and edification. They avoided losing their identity and becoming alienated. They also transformed their disillusionment in everything and everyone—including themselves—into writings that can seize a reader many generations later. The power of their words helped them to rise above their internal inferno, so that they could stay, at least for a time, in purgatory—not to mention the possibility of reaching paradise. But they were not really, however, travelers through hell. Only those who have experienced the ultimate degradation of humanity have truly experienced hell.They have stood so often in the doorway leading to their almost certain death that they have lost count. But miraculously, some have remained with us. I have met one of those travelers.

Vancouver, Spring 1987

I am sitting face to face with Rudolf Vrba, whom I have previously seen only on the screen in Claude Lanzmann's monumental film "Shoah." In that film, Vrba described his time in Auschwitz between 1942 and 1944. He was at first an ordinary death camp prisoner, but eventually he was promoted to the position of registrar, giving him a certain degree of freedom of movement and a general familiarity with the camp.

Vrba's answers to Lanzmann's questions were composed and matter-of-fact, with an extraordinary detachment frequently accompanied by a sardonic smile. I cannot forget the expression on Vrba's face as he explained the difference between Auschwitz and the other concentration camps, many of which maintained a more or less stable population of prisoners to provide labor for the German war industry. The camp at Mauthausen, for instance, was used to quarry stone. Auschwitz was also a kind of factory, but its main product was death.

Lanzmann moved from one interview subject to another with the unperturbable reassurance of a detached analyst. Vrba was followed by another remarkable survivor, Filip Müller, who had been a member of the *Sonderkommando*, the prisoner group responsible for the "dirty work" at the gas chambers and the crematorium—removing the bodies. These workers were themselves also eventually executed. The conversation with Vrba then resumed. It was impossible to imagine anything worse than the horror of the tales these two were telling. And yet they went on to describe one episode after another, each more gruesome than the one before.

In his last interview with Lanzmann, Vrba described the gassing of the so-called family camp, whose inhabitants had been transported to Auschwitz from the model ghetto camp at Theresienstadt. Contrary to the usual routine at Auschwitz, the families were permitted to stay together for six months, only to be gassed suddenly. The killings were particularly violent and ruthless, if one might be allowed to use such inadequate words in such a context. Vrba had known about the impending doom through his contacts as camp registrar. When he saw the first indications, he was able to contact a small resistance group that, against all odds, continued to function in the camp. The group was headed by the non-Jewish political prisoners who had a somewhat privileged position among all the prisoners. They tried to organize a revolt in the family camp, but it never came about. The resistance movement had selected the camp's teacher, Freddy Hirsch, to organize the revolt, but Hirsch preferred instead to commit suicide, because he did not want to hasten the inevitable killing of the schoolchildren.

After the liquidation of the family camp, Vrba chose a different and, according to all odds, equally hopeless avenue. He and a fellow countryman from Slovakia, Fred Wetzler, decided to escape. All previous attempts at escape had failed and had led to torture and execution in front of all of the camp's inmates. But Vrba and Wetzler succeeded, becoming the first ever to flee Auschwitz. Their remarkable escape has been described in detail.[1]

At first they hid in a lumberyard in the area between the outer and inner fences of the camp. They lay completely still for several days while the SS searched for them intensively. To keep the SS dogs away, they smeared themselves with poor-quality tobacco drenched with kerosene. The historian Martin Gilbert has described the extraordinary efforts made by the SS to capture them.[2] Gestapo headquarters in Berlin put all security units, criminal police, and border patrol stations in the eastern region on alert. Himmler was kept informed. After several days of searching, the SS concluded that the two had succeeded in their escape and discontinued the hunt inside the camp itself. After many long, dangerous nights wandering on foot without any identification documents, a compass or map, or any weapons or money, they finally reached their homeland, Slovakia.

Their escape took on major historical significance because it provided the first eyewitness account from the largest of the death camps. Current historical accounts refer to it simply as "The Auschwitz Report."

In the film, Vrba told Lanzmann that he decided to escape in order to warn the largest surviving Jewish community under Hitler's occupation, the Hungarian Jews. He hoped to incite them to revolt rather than submit to being deported. In his role as registrar, Vrba knew that the Germans were preparing Auschwitz for a speedy annihilation of the Hungarian Jews who had, until then, been relatively unharmed. As early as several months before Germany's invasion of Hungary on March 19, 1944, a new crematorium and new railroad tracks had been built at Auschwitz. The SS troops joked about the "Hungarian salami" that they were looking forward to.

Some weeks after Vrba and Wetzler arrived in Slovakia, their report reached the Allied governments. It was also distributed to leaders of the Jewish communities in Hungary and other countries. But in the film Vrba says, with a feeling of resignation, that it didn't do very much good.

In a review of "Shoah" in the *New York Times* on November 3, 1980, Elie Wiesel calls Vrba "an authentic hero," but he admits that he is afraid to meet him. He dreads the question, "Why did you allow yourself to be deported to Auschwitz? Didn't I warn you?"

It was immediately clear to me that the report I had been given to read under a promise of secrecy in Budapest in May 1944—at the age of nineteen and at a time when deportations from the Hungarian countryside were at their peak—was identical to the Auschwitz report of Vrba and Wetzler. As I listened to Vrba, I was reminded of the dry, matter-of-fact language of the report, but the abstract had suddenly found a face and a voice, now speaking to me from the screen. The entire span of forty-three years was blown away, and I was filled with the same mixture of nausea and a degree of intellectual satisfaction with its relentless logic that I felt then. Even as I read the report for the first time, it was evident to me that it represented the horrors of reality rather than the many unrealistic lies and self-deceiving excuses that we had previously been fed from so many different sources.

I decided to try to find Vrba and tell him of what enormous help his report had been to me. If I had not known what was awaiting me at the other end of the train trip, I would never have dared to risk an escape.

It was not difficult to find Vrba, for it turned out that we were scientific colleagues. He is a professor of neuropharmacology in Vancouver, and I am now sitting in a comfortable armchair in the faculty club at a Canadian university, talking with someone who, at first glance, seems quite ordinary. He impresses me as being relaxed and jovial. By now I have also read his book, and I am aware that he has survived more death sentences than anyone else I have ever met. He has also witnessed more human evil, more closely, more profoundly, and for a longer period of time than any other survivor I know. Only the dead could have more to tell.

Vrba's book was very difficult reading, despite its successful outcome. I had to take it in very small doses, two or three pages only now and then—and absolutely never in the evenings. The best time was during a busy workday, when retreat from the planet of Auschwitz to the reality of the moment was ensured. At the same time I felt an irresistible urge to read his book and other eyewitness reports. I wanted to keep Auschwitz, this universe of death, in my sight and remember how it could operate in this century, not far from here. But why? Was it to honor my murdered family, my murdered classmates? Or was it rather to steel myself against the darkest side of our human heritage?

I ask Vrba why the new edition of his book is called *Escape from Auschwitz*, while the first edition, published in 1964, was entitled *I Cannot Forgive*. "What was it that you could not forgive?"

Vrba answers with his sardonic smile, "I don't want to tell you that. The Hungarian-English writer George Mikes has also been wondering a great deal about the same question. But I haven't told him either."[3]

I could think of several possible explanations. The mass murders of the Nazis were so obvious that no further comments were needed. But Vrba's enigmatic title might mean much more. It could refer to the failure of the Allies to bomb the crematoria in Auschwitz or the railways leading there, despite the fact that it was completely obvious what was going on. He might also be referring to the Jewish leaders in Hungary, whom he has criticized bitterly for failing to warn the Jewish population and urging them to resist. A well-known Zionist leader in Budapest, Dr. Kastner, had read the report but, according to Vrba, decided to keep its contents secret in return for a promise by the Germans of safety for sixteen-hundred people, to be selected by Kastner. The group was to include his family, young Zionists, and wealthy Jews who paid for their safety with gold and other valuables that Eichmann needed to pay for "the German war effort."

I didn't agree at all with Vrba on this point, because I had seen Kastner at work during the period. His headquarters were at the Jewish Council, previously called the Jewish Community Office, in Budapest. I was working there, first as an errand boy and later as secretary to one of the members of the council. I knew that Kastner was trying to select a number of people for rescue, but that I had no chance of being included in that privileged group. Nevertheless, he was a hero in my eyes, and he remained so in the years that followed. He rescued many while the rest of us tried to save only ourselves or, at best, the members of our families. Kastner's activities became the subject of a libel case in Israel during the 1950s. It began when Kastner sued a relatively obscure journalist named Malchier Greenwald, who had written an article in a Hungarian-language Israeli newspaper accusing Kastner of collaboration with the Nazis. The case went to trial in May 1953. In its first decision in 1955, the court acquitted Greenwald of libel. Then, on March 3, 1957, Kastner was murdered on the street by a deranged young man whose family had been killed by the Nazis. In January of 1958, the Supreme Court of Israel reconsidered the original case and, by a split vote of three to two, convicted Greenwald. Kastner had finally won.

The process aroused very intense reactions in Israel, and feelings are polarized to this day. But my own conversations with many people have convinced me that Kastner's position is much better understood and appreciated now than it was earlier. The division of opinion is also reflected in the Supreme Court decision of 1958 and the controversy that it generated. One of the judges who voted against the majority opinion concluded that Kastner had entered into a pact with the devil himself. The President of the Court, Justice Agranat, was of a quite different opinion. His lengthy introduction to the written decision begins with a crystal-clear historical analysis of the circumstances that prevailed in Budapest in 1944, quoting the Biblical interpreter, Rabbi Hillel: "Judge not thy neighbor until thou art in his place."

I pointed out to Vrba that the publication of his report could not have led to a massive general uprising as he had wished. My own experience serves as an example. I had read the report a few weeks after it was prepared. It was one of the first copies prepared from the original that Kastner and the other members of the Jewish Council had received. My supervisor gave me permission to tell my relatives and close friends about the report so that they could go underground in time. Of the dozen or so people I warned, not one believed me.

But that was exactly the problem, answered Vrba. Why were the contents of the report distributed only through private circles and in such secrecy? Why had the Jewish Council not blared their warnings loudly and openly for all? Why was the report not published for general circulation? Why did your leaders not urge you to rebel? You were a mere boy—why would anyone believe what you were saying? The Jews would certainly have believed their responsible leaders.

I answered skeptically that I didn't believe that the majority of the Jews in Budapest were ready to see the terrible truth. There might have been a few, but certainly not the majority. Vrba himself makes exactly that point in his book when he describes the reactions of those already in Auschwitz, who could see it with their own eyes. Primo Levi and others have described how otherwise sensible and logical people could explain away the black smoke that spewed from the chimneys of the crematoria, the horrible odor of burnt human flesh. Miklós Nyiszli, the Hungarian Jewish pathologist and Mengele's forced assistant, describes how prisoners, who knew full well that no one ever returned from the gas chambers, repressed such knowledge as they themselves lined up for execution in front of the chamber doors.[4] Besides, why are you so bitter about what didn't or couldn't happen in Hungary in 1944? Why are you not more satisfied and proud of your own achievements? The report by you and Wetzler was largely responsible for the fact that the Pope and the king of Sweden appealed to the Hungarian Regent Miklós Horthy, and that President Roosevelt gave his famous speech declaring the punishment that would await the war criminals. Because of these interventions and Mrs. Horthy's reaction to the report, Horthy intervened and stopped the deportations on July 7, only one week before the remainder of the Hungarian Jews, the two-hundred thousand Jews of Budapest, were scheduled to join the eight-hundred thousand from the provinces who had already gone to their end in the gas chambers during Eichmann's "blitz operation" of May and June. Shouldn't you be satisfied that you managed to save two-hundred thousand?

No, Vrba was not satisfied. He saw his glass half empty, not half full. I did not agree with him, but what right did I have to tell him so? Nevertheless, I tried.

"It was relatively easy for me to believe your report. I was young and vigorous and had nothing to lose. Nevertheless, I hesitated until the very last moment. It was not until I saw the freight cars in front of me that I had the courage to run, despite the risk of being shot. But what more could you have expected from a law-abiding citizen, the head of a family, unprepared suddenly to change his opinion of a government that had until that time been reasonably respectable—to recognize it for the gang of criminals it had become, to expose his children to the risk of being gunned down? If you really harbored greater expectations, you were completely unrealistic. As long as families were able to stay together, especially if they were in their own homes, such thoughts were unbearable for most of them. Denial, the idea that 'it couldn't be that bad,' was therefore quite natural."

Vrba shook his head. "You are ignoring the most important fact! The whole Nazi program of annihilation was based on lies, deceptive rumors, and hellishly clever traps. The leaders of the Jewish community responded by disseminating reassuring and misleading information instead of speaking out in plain language, warning and organizing a last-ditch rebellion. That might have amounted to no more than suicide, as great or greater than the revolt in the Warsaw ghetto. Many would have died, but far fewer than in Auschwitz. And they would have perished with their dignity intact."

"No, I don't agree at all," I replied. "The Jewish leaders whom I knew were no heros, but they tried to do whatever they could in that desperate situation. They appealed and warned, they tried to find a way out or, at least, a temporary respite. Their only alternative was to commit suicide, like Czerniakowski, the president of the Jewish Council in Warsaw or like your own friend, the teacher that you mentioned in the Lanzmann film. Even the president of the Jewish Council in Budapest, Samuel Stern, committed suicide at the end."

"No," said Vrba, still shaking his head. We changed the subject.

"How can you live and function in this pleasant, friendly, and rather provincial place where no one has the slightest concept of what you went through?" I asked him. "How can anyone who has experienced all that you have described in your book still sit quietly, making small talk with waiters or colleagues? I know other survivors of Auschwitz who have quite successfully repressed their memories and who manage very well, at least until the nightmares reappear suddenly. But you must go back constantly to those days. You are called in as a witness at trials of old Nazis or their followers, people who claim that the holocaust never happened. You try to describe something that cannot be described in any human language, you try to explain the incomprehensible, you want people to listen to something they do not want to hear. How can you keep your sanity? By the way, have you been back to Auschwitz since the war?"

"Yes, I have," he said impassively. "Ten years after I escaped, I attended a conference in Poland. A bus tour was arranged to Auschwitz, and I went along."

"How did you react? Did you tell your colleagues what you had experienced there?"

"No. I didn't even mention that I had ever been to Auschwitz before."

"But why not?"

"What would have been the use? No one who has not experienced it can understand. None of the many books ever written about it, not even my book, could convey the sense of what it was really like. Lanzmann's film was the first fairly successful attempt to approach the subject, to listen to the voices of the survivors, to hear their silence, to dare to look into their faces."

"But do any of your colleagues, your assistants, your Canadian friends, know what you have experienced?"

At first Vrba did not answer. Then, with an odd smile, he said that one of his colleagues became very upset when he quite unexpectedly saw Vrba in Lanzmann's film. He wondered if all the horrible things that Vrba described in the film were really true.

"I do not know," Vrba answered. "I was only an actor reciting my lines."

"How strange," the colleague remarked. "I didn't know that you were an actor. Why did they say that film was made without any actors?"

I was speechless. Only now did I understand that this was the same man who lay quiet and motionless for three days in the hollow pile of lumber while Auschwitz was on maximum alert, only a few yards from the armed SS men and their dogs combing the area so thoroughly. If he could do that, then he certainly could also don the mask of a professor and manage everyday conversation with his colleagues in Vancouver, in Canada, that paradise land that is never fully appreciated by its own citizens, a people without the slightest notion of the planet Auschwitz. Neither the children of paradise nor the children of hell can dissociate themselves altogether from their own worlds. It is only a few rare individuals who make courageous attempts to penetrate the unbearable occasionally, but they cannot venture out too far from the well-protected spaceships of their own psychology either.

Do I dare approach the planet Auschwitz? My own space capsule is circling in an orbit closer than that of my Canadian or Swedish colleagues to that horrible world, but it is still much farther away than Vrba's orbit. What I experienced in Nazi-occupied Budapest compared with Vrba's experience at Auschwitz is like a shampoo at the barber shop compared with decapitation by a guillotine.

After ten hours of almost uninterrupted conversation, we parted like old friends despite the differences in our views. I hoped to see him again soon, but I was also longing to forget about him, not to have to think about what he can and cannot forgive. But I knew that I would never be able to forget his sardonic smile.

Los Angeles, Summer 1987

From Vancouver I continued on to a symposium in California, where I was scheduled to give a talk. During the lunch break, I sat next to one of my former graduate students, now a professor at the university. We talked like old friends—the years had completely disappeared. But suddenly he changed the subject. He told me that he had met an apparently pleasant and intelligent Austrian colleague in his forties, who declared after a few drinks that the gassing of millions of Jews never actually took place. The Austrian talked about the "big Jewish lie" that he had uncovered through his own "research." He was convinced that the Jews had fabricated this myth to coerce the world into giving them a nation of their own. He claimed that the myth was created in collusion with the CIA and the Soviet Union after the Second World War. He declared that even the "Waldheim affair" was a typical fabrication concocted by the tireless work of the worldwide Jewish conspiracy. It was merely the latest link in the chain of efforts to maintain the illusion of the holocaust. During his very emotional monologue, the Austrian pointed out time and again that he was not anti-Semitic. On the contrary, many of his friends were Jewish.

My colleague, who was born several years after the war, was so amazed that he didn't know what to say, especially since he was just about to leave to catch a plane. Because of the rapid pace of the discussion and the generally friendly atmosphere, he could not come up with an appropriate answer to what he perceived to be absurd and classically anti-Semitic remarks, even though they had been presented with such great certainty. He felt somewhat like a traitor and asked if I could recommend anything for him to read in order to be better prepared the next time.

How, indeed, could one answer that question? What literature should one give to someone having to confront people so thoroughly convinced by their own irrational arguments, whether they concern the holocaust, supernatural powers, living cells that they think have been produced in test tubes, or deadly viruses produced by the Pentagon? Is it possible to use rational arguments to counter such profound delusions?

I thought of SS officer Suchomel in Lanzmann's film, photographed by a hidden camera, describing the last hour of the women standing naked in below-zero temperature in the underground tunnel leading to the gas chambers of Treblinka. He talked of their anxiety when they realized that their death was coming, as they heard the screams of the men who had preceded them into the gas chambers and understood that they were merely waiting their turn. I remember his composed, dispassionate, and monotonous voice, describing in gruesome detail how the women lost control of their bodily functions. I was seized by a rage that I could barely suppress, but because it was time for my lecture, I could not allow myself to yield to that feeling.

An hour of concentrating on cells, chromosomes, and cancer genes reestablished my peace of mind. It was time for questions and then a coffee break. Suddenly I saw two women, one young and the other elderly, who seemed to be very eager to talk to me. The older woman spoke with a strong Hungarian accent and mentioned my father's name. I changed immediately to my mother tongue. She told me that she and I used to play together on my grandmother's farm when I was eleven years old and she was six. She described the farm, the outhouse, the vegetable garden, the stable, and our favorite playground, the big haystacks. It was correct to every detail, just like a photograph. I asked her daughter with the long black hair whether she understood our conversation. She replied in Hungarian overlaid with a strong

American accent. She turned out to be studying engineering. How did they manage to find me? The daughter had noticed my name on the bulletin board. She had previously heard that I was alive and living in Stockholm.

I asked the mother if she had remained in my father's village even during her teenage years. No, she lived in a nearby town. What happened in 1944? "Auschwitz," she answered.

An assistant returned my slides from the lecture and another colleague asked if I would mind taking some cells back to Stockholm with me.

"How did you manage to survive?" I asked.

"A man from the *Sonderkommando* who met us at the unloading platform in Auschwitz warned me to lie about my age. I told them I was eighteen instead of fourteen. That saved my life."

A departmental secretary interrupted our conversation. I had to sign some papers to arrange to be reimbursed for my travel expenses.

"Did you know you were in Auschwitz? Did you know about the gas chambers?"

"Yes and no. My father had previously met some Polish refugees who told him some of the facts. When he was forced to pack up his most valuable possessions, he insisted on taking his prayer shawl and the other religious items without which no orthodox Jew would ever take a step, even though he knew that he would have no use for them where he was going. We believed him, but we also didn't believe him."

Again a colleague interrupted and asked if I would please send his greetings to a good friend in Stockholm.

"What happened to your father?"

"He went to the gas chamber. Mengele himself made the selection. He arrived at the train platform on his motorbike and seemed very polite. He looked at my mother, who was forty-two and very beautiful, and said, 'You can still work.' She went off to the right and stood in the same line where I was standing. But suddenly she saw her little four-year-old nephew, who had apparently been separated from his mother and was wandering about. My mother took hold of the boy's hand. Mengele was already sitting on his motorbike, ready to speed off, when he too noticed the boy. He got off his bike, came back to the line, grabbed a cane from an old man, put the crook of the cane around my mother's neck, pulled her and the boy out of the line and moved them to the other line on the left, the one leading straight to the gas chamber. I never saw her again."

She spoke calmly, as if talking about an ordinary event of everyday life in Los Angeles the previous week.

I was interrupted by yet another colleague, who introduced me to a student. They were telling me about an experiment they thought would interest me. Then my scientific host appeared. He had been worried about the intrusion of the two strange women and suspected that they were trying to "monopolize" me. I felt that I owed him some sort of explanation, and I introduced the older woman, explaining that she was on the same deportation train to Auschwitz as my grandmother and my uncles, none of whom ever returned. My colleague stared at me, groping for words, obviously not knowing what to say. I have often noticed this same reaction. Indeed, what could one really say? He left.

"Do you remember my grandmother?"

"Oh, do I! I loved Aunti Fáni. My own grandmother was also called Fáni. She also ended her life in the gas chamber. She was as devoted to her family as your grandmother was."

What would the Austrian have said? Surely he would have found an answer somewhere among his preconceived notions.

The secretary approached again. Politely, she reminded me that there were others who wanted to talk to me. "Yes, I'm coming. I'll be right there."

Paris, Fall 1987

We were three apparently quite ordinary people, strolling among the crowd on the Boulevard St. Michel on a beautiful Saturday afternoon. We soaked up the autumn sun as we ambled along through the fallen leaves in the Jardin de Luxembourg, watching the many colorful young people around us. But we didn't really pay much attention to them. For a while, we continued along the banks of the Seine, and then we turned around and headed toward the Latin Quarter, where we spent some more time sitting in cafés, ordering, paying, and talking, seemingly relaxed like everyone else. But in reality our minds were elsewhere, as far from

Paris as possible. We had traveled from different places and come together to descend voluntarily to hell. One of us, Benno Müller-Hill, was a German molecular biologist who had taken a sabbatical leave from his experiments to carry on his historical research on the role of the German scientists in the mass murders of psychiatric patients, Jews, and gypsies.[5] I myself, who had at one time stood next to the inferno and experienced the horror of having a large part of my family annihilated, had managed to escape. The third was Vrba, the traveler through hell.

Earlier that afternoon I had brought together my two newfound friends. Vrba was in Paris to brush up on his French and check the translation of his book. Benno had come to Paris to visit his colleagues at the Pasteur Institute and also to meet Vrba. I was traveling through Paris after a scientific meeting in Lyon.

Who was living closer to reality, the young people strolling around the Latin Quarter, or the three of us?

I had a strong sense of unreality as we waited for the traffic light to change in front of the Café Dupont and as we crowded together with the tourists at Notre Dame. The enormous facade of the cathedral was there in front of us, but this time it looked almost like a kitsch theater set. Vrba suggested that we visit the holocaust memorial behind Notre Dame.

That walk of only a few minutes took us from the noisy tourist crowd to the silence of the museum's rooms, where you feel alone and isolated among the symbolic chains and barbed wire. A faint glow of sunlight came in through the narrow openings in the wall. We were surrounded by the voices of the victims, forcing themselves upon us from all the inscriptions on the walls pressing in around us, as if they wanted to drink our sacrificial blood. They reminded me of the shadows that surrounded Odysseus when he visited Hades to ask Teiresias, the wise seer, how he might find his way home.

The outer courtyard of the memorial was surrounded by a wall that ended with a sharp point at the east side of the Ile de la Cité. The narrow, slanted openings of the wall pointed downward. The much-celebrated city had vanished as though it had never existed. The water swirled and flowed toward an unidentifiable and inexorable eternity. The walls towered above, turning away from us and yet simultaneously closing in. We were in the chamber of death.

We were all completely speechless. Even Vrba's macabre sense of humor and his sharp sarcasm had fallen silent for the moment.

Some time later we found ourselves sitting in a small bistro. I asked Vrba what he thought of Benno's conclusion that the German anthropologists, human geneticists, and psychiatrists had laid the ideological groundwork for the Nazi mass murders— that they were the architects of the holocaust, not merely passive followers. Benno had concluded from his exhaustive documentation that, contrary to what many wanted so desperately to believe, the "euthanasia programs" of the mental hospitals and the horrible human experiments with the "valuable scientific material" from Auschwitz, as Mengele described it, could not be ascribed to a small minority of madmen, opportunists, or charlatans. On the contrary, they had been carried out by quite ordinary—and in some instances, eminent—physicians and scientists.

Vrba was not particularly convinced by this interpretation. He thought that the ideology of race biology might have played a minor role, but that would not explain why so many apparently ordinary people took part in the murders without showing any signs of remorse, or how the annihilation program could have been carried out with such efficiency. He thought that some other factors must have been far more important. His views were shaped strongly by his own period of imprisonment, during which he worked in a section of Auschwitz called "Canada." This was the commercial center of the camp, a kind of giant department store where hundreds of prisoners worked sorting, registering, and packing clothes, foodstuffs, valuables, and other goods and property taken from the prisoners on their way to the gas chambers.[6] There certainly was a lot of it, because the Jews often wanted to bring their most valued possessions in the hope that they might be of some use later. In the words of the official propaganda, the deportation of the Jews was part of a "resettlement," as if they were merely changing homes.

"Canada" was a large square yard surrounded by barbed wire, with a watchtower in each corner, enclosing several enormous storage buildings. In a special section were all the valuables—cash, gold, jewelry, and precious stones. There were huge piles of suitcases, blankets, children's clothing, fur coats, baby carriages, and women's hair, all waiting for distribution and processing. One report sent to Himmler on February 6, 1943, stated that by that date, the camp had sent back to Germany 825 truckloads containing 97,000 men's suits, 76,000 dresses, 132,000 shirts, 155,000 coats, three tons of woman's hair, enormous amounts of children's clothing, $50,000 in cash, and gold valued at $116,420.

Vrba's experiences in "Canada" made him more inclined to ascribe economic motives to the mass murders. Otherwise, why did the murders start in 1941 and not in 1939, when war broke out? Vrba thought that might be explained by the war situation in the fall of 1941. At that time leading generals of the *Wehrmacht* began to realize that Hitler's blitzkrieg against the Soviet Union was about to go amiss, and that they would have to count on a long, drawn-out war on the eastern front. That would leave Germany's western defense system weakened in the event of campaigns there.[7] Large contingents of the German army were kept tied up in the occupied countries. That was a great burden to the war effort. Increasingly they had to rely on local collaborators, or "quislings." The local Nazis were the obvious candidates, but their services were costly. They could not be paid in German currency, so weakened by the war. The Jews of Europe had hard currency, gold, and jewelry, but it wouldn't have been nearly enough simply to take it from the Jews. The quislings had to be reassured that the Jews would never come back.

According to Vrba, the driving forces for the Nazis were greed and the desire for a comfortable life. Vrba saw many signs of this among the SS personnel in Auschwitz. Nobody had to work in the camp against his will. A simple request for transfer was always granted, even if it usually meant service at the front. But the "bourgeois have a tendency to go berserk whenever they can satisfy their own avarice," Vrba said, and he proceeded to illustrate his point with a series of harrowing anecdotes. I will recount only one such episode. A non-Jewish doctor, Ella Lingens-Reinert, who became an assistant minister of health in Austria after the war, was sent to Auschwitz for having harbored a Jew in her home in Vienna. As a non-Jewish prisoner, she had a privileged position and was respected even by the SS women. One day she was standing with an SS woman whose husband also worked at Auschwitz, watching a long line of children, women, and old or incapacitated men waiting in front of the gas chamber. She asked the SS woman, "Do you like working here?" "No, Frau Doktor," answered the woman, "I don't really like it." "But then why do you do it? You could be transferred if you wanted." "Yes, but you see, it is like this. My husband and I both come from very simple families, we are hard-working people, and for many years we have been hoping to live in a better area. We want to have pleasant and respectable neighbors and friends. It is only now that we have been able to buy a house in a nice suburb. It is almost ready, but the kitchen is still far from finished. If we work here for only six more months, we can have it finished and then invite our neighbors. Then we will stop working here."

No, she did not like her job, but the kitchen was far more important.

Vrba had a similar interpretation of the work of the SS doctors. The racist ideology that culminated in the relegation of Jews to a class of subhuman beings was an important prerequisite for the program of annihilation. But that alone cannot explain why so many doctors remained in their positions in Auschwitz for so long and participated in the murders with such equanimity. The diary of SS physician Paul Kremer, one of the documents presented at the Nuremberg trials, is especially enlightening in this context.[8] Kremer was in the SS reserves and started his service at Auschwitz when he was already fifty-nine years old. He remained there for only several months, but long enough to be placed in charge of the killings and to take an active part in the death of 10,717 people between September 2 and November 8, 1942. He was a gastroenterologist and an unsuccessful scientist, with dubious theories that had not received recognition in the German academic world. He had become frustrated and bitter. But he loved good food, a glass of cognac, and good conversation with educated friends. All these things he found at Auschwitz. In his meticulously thorough diary, he often describes small enjoyable events and the pleasant company at the SS club next to the concentration camp. It is only in passing that he mentions the "special actions (*Sonderaktion*)," the official euphemistic code name for the executions, in which he took part. In one entry he writes that Dante's inferno is nothing compared to this place. In another note, he calls Auschwitz the anus of the world. The "special action" against the "Musulmanen," the camp's most severely emaciated prisoners, was in his words the "most horrible of the horrible." But, he added, the SS men participated willingly in these actions because they received an extra-large ration of schnapps, cigarettes, and sausage.

Kremer writes much more about his own minor ailments than about his "work." He returns constantly to his "outstanding dinners" and notes the menus for most of them. He is particular about the brand of mineral water and praises the desserts, especially *das herrliche Vanilleneis* (the magnificent vanilla ice cream). With the next stroke of his pen he describes naked Jewish women who beg for their lives, in vain—"*entsetzlich!*" (terrible!) But most of the time the entries simply state *Sonderaktion*, with a note of the time and date but no other details. At one point he notes briefly that he provided medical assistance at a thrashing and a "small arms execution." Immediately thereafter he turns to notes on his daily ration of soap. He also writes about his measurements that he sent to a tailor in Berlin when he ordered a new uniform. He praises the prisoners' orchestra—the conductor is from the State Opera in Warsaw! After the concert, he ate "*Schweinebraten. Es gab echten Bohnenkaffee, ausgezeichnetes Bier und belegte Brötchen!*" (Roast pork. There was real coffee, wonderful beer, and sandwiches!)

There isn't much about Kremer's "research," but he writes repeatedly that he obtains absolutely fresh material from newly executed prisoners. At the Nuremberg trials, he described how his "patients" were placed on the post mortem table, alive. He asked them about the symptoms and diseases that interested him. The autopsy assistant then injected fatal doses of phenol directly into the heart as Kremer stood ready with his instruments, so that he could get his material for fixation in only a few seconds. Toward the end of the diary, Kremer expresses horror at the Anglo-American bombings of Germany. "They bomb even the churches!" he exclaims. "How far can humans go in their barbarism? If they attack cultural monuments, they make war on the whole of civilized humanity, not only on us. My heart writhes with pain when I see such things. How can God allow these buildings, made to honor his glory, to be so completely destroyed?"

Of all the SS doctors at Auschwitz, Vrba pointed out that Benno focused his attention mostly on Mengele. That might be because Mengele was a student of the two professors who had originated the theory of race biology, Professors Fischer and Verschuer at the Kaiser Wilhelm Institute for Anthropology in Berlin. In Mengele, Müller-Hill sees the prototype for the perverted, ideologically motivated scientist who wants to "purify the Aryan race." But Vrba was more skeptical of the ideological motivation, even in the case of Mengele. As we know, he had delivered fixed brains and other tissues from the victims to many prominent professors in the German academic system. The recipients were fully aware of the source of the material and had given exact instructions for the preparation, preservation, and transportation of the tissues. According to Vrba, Mengele wanted to ingratiate himself with the prominent professors to foster his own academic career. He had no loftier goals, not even perverted ones. He was merely a small-time climber, but one who did not hesitate to murder.

The discussions between Benno and Vrba continued for several hours. At first they took diametrically opposed positions, but after a while they began slowly to agree with one another. Finally they concluded that they were both correct. The concepts of racial ideology had provided justification for mass murder, and the criminal government had sanctioned, implemented, and institutionalized it. Within the perverted universe of the death camp, one could discover all the motivations that existed in the society at large, but in the camps the images were distorted, as in a convex mirror. If Mengele was the perverted researcher driven to establish his academic career, then Kremer represented the type of doctor who chose medicine as a route toward creature comforts and a high standard of living.

In his foreword to *Commandant in Auschwitz*, the memoirs written by the Auschwitz base commander Rudolf Höss, the Norwegian author Arnulf Øverland writes, "From the technical and quantitative point of view, his (Höss's) crimes exceed everything in the world history of mass murders. Nevertheless, this autobiography demonstrates that, in most respects, Höss was indistinguishable from ordinary human beings. That is precisely what makes his book one of the most horrible in the history of literature." Exactly the same might be said for most of the other Nazi doctors.[9]

All German doctors had taken the Hippocratic oath and sworn to heal, ease suffering, and provide comfort. Could it be that these sacred promises, the core of our proud tradition of Western culture, have so quickly been stripped of all their meaning and become no more than shallow formalities? Or has the gradual shallowing merely been pushed to its extreme logical consequence in this case?

Later that evening we were invited for dinner with François Jacob, one of the principal pioneers of modern molecular biology. In addition to his Nobel Prize-winning scientific work, Jacob is also well known as a writer. His first great work, *La Logique du Vivant*, deals with the development of concepts of biology since the sixteenth century. His collection of essays, *The Possible and the Actual*, examines the logic of scientific reasoning and the ways in which scientists work. Jacob's recently published autobiography, *The Statue Within*, has been praised as one of the best—if not the best—autobiography ever written by a scientist. The book describes the birth of some of this century's most important biological discoveries, arising from the interaction among the unique trio of scientists at the Pasteur Institute, André Lwoff, Jacques Monod, and François Jacob—three very different men with two decades of age difference between them. But Jacob's book deals with much more than the history of science. His childhood, his escape from German-occupied France, and his wartime exploits as one of General De Gaulle's most highly decorated soldiers in the African campaign were previously practically unknown, even to his friends and colleagues.

I have known Jacob for more than thirty years. He is not a facile conversationalist—just the opposite. He prefers to listen to others and talk very little. This is partly due to the thousands of shrapnel pieces that he has carried in his body since the war. They cause him pain, particularly when the weather is about to change. He always finds it difficult to sit still for prolonged periods of time. When he is a bit disinterested, he seems completely absent. If he does become involved in a conversation, he makes short comments and asks only simple questions. Some people who do not like Jacob find him thoroughly boring. But in his autobiography, Jacob the writer and storyteller has painted a completely different picture of himself. The book is characterized by an unusual sense of intensity and vitality. The narrator is both participant and observer, present and absent at the same time, sensitive but aloof, abstract and indifferent, yet concrete and vital.

The meeting with Jacob was arranged at my initiative. I was a bit worried as we climbed the stairs to his apartment in the Latin Quarter. What would happen if my friends didn't like each other?

It didn't go so badly after all. After a glass of sherry at Jacob's home, we went to a small restaurant around the corner where Jacob is a regular customer. At first we talked about some mutual friends, and then took on, or at least pretended to take on, the air of seriousness associated with ordering dinner in a French restaurant.

Jacob asked Vrba why he had come to Paris. Vrba said that his book describing his escape from Auschwitz was being translated into French and he was proofreading the manuscript. He was also taking a crash course in French at the Sorbonne. In the middle of all this work, however, he also was asked to take on yet another obligation. The ultra-right leader Le Pen had recently declared that the annihilation of the Jews should be viewed as only one of many episodes of the war, and he even questioned whether the gas chambers ever existed.

The French radio service had asked Vrba to respond to these statements, and he showed us the text of his proposed comments. They were crystal clear, as long as one didn't choose to turn a deaf ear to them. But that is exactly what a small but steadily increasing segment of humanity was preparing to do. Vrba described the many figures in the United States, Canada, France, and other countries who have chosen to forge history. In Sweden, Radio Islam broadcasts classically anti-Semitic programs, asserting that the holocaust never took place and accusing the Jews, in conspiracy with Zionists and Bolsheviks, of having invented it. One of the American "revisionists" was R.A. Butz, who had been a rather mediocre and obscure researcher in a low-level position at Northwestern University in Chicago. After being "converted" by the French instigator of the revisionist theories, Faurrisson, he

suddenly became something of a celebrity. Since then, the denial
of history has become his life's work. His basic premise is that the
myth of Auschwitz was created by no less than Vrba himself.
According to Butz, Vrba was an incompetent youngster, a lazy
troublemaker in whom the good German authorities wanted to
instill the work ethic. With this as their underlying positive,
educational motivation, they sent him to a work camp called
Auschwitz. But Vrba was not able, even there, to keep a job, and
he chose to escape. After being paid by the Zionists, the CIA , and
the Bolsheviks, he collaborated with these organizations to con-
coct the myth about Auschwitz.

I asked Vrba if it was possible to sue these people. Yes, it was
possible, but the expenses of a lawsuit could become enormous.
Furthermore, because of the laws protecting freedom of speech,
it was often very difficult to win such cases and to prove the
defendants guilty. The enemies of democracy have often abused
the rights guaranteed by it to pursue their own nefarious goals.
But there is in Canada a law that prohibits interference with the
rightful and legitimate grieving of another person. Through use
of this law, a woman who had lost her parents in the gas chambers
of Auschwitz brought suit against the Canadian representative of
the revisionist movement. After a legal process that lasted many
years, the accused was found guilty in a lower court. However,
because of legal technicalities, the verdict was overturned by a
higher appeals court. The case must now be heard again, and the
costs will be astronomical.

Who in the world would listen to these latter-day followers of
Joseph Goebbels, whose main thesis was that a lie becomes the
truth if it is repeated often enough?

There is, according to Vrba, an unholy alliance between the
classical, rabid anti-Semites who wish to wash clean the record of
Nazism, and more "moderate" anti-Semites who think that Jews
have been complaining far too much. To these two groups might
be added the political anti-Zionists that come in a variety of anti-
Semitic shades and wish only to promote their own goals. Many
are opportunists like the scientific charlatans of cancer research
and other fields, people who do not hesitate to deny even the most
well-documented facts if it suits their personal ambitions. But the
heresy of charlatans can assume validity only when planted in the

fertile soil of widespread wishful thinking. Generations that have not experienced persecutions and discrimination, totalitarianism, or foreign occupation want very much to believe that man is basically good and incapable of atrocities of such a magnitude. Even if one were to accept the historical facts, it is often convenient to blame the Nazi war crimes on a small handful of madmen, thereby ignoring the fact that Hitler attained the office of Chancellor of the Reich through an entirely lawful process. Often one does not want to admit that most of the mass murderers were quite ordinary people. Others are willing to admit the facts of the past, but wish to put the past completely behind them and ignore it altogether. The movement, promulgated by Nolte, to relegate the holocaust to the role of just another historical incident is one good example of this approach. The Nazi programs and the suppression of memory are wrapped in academic attire, and the organized mass murders are viewed in their historical perspective merely as one of the many tragic occurrences of war. Parallels are drawn to the role of mass acquiescence during the purges of the Stalin era in the Soviet Union. Hitler is seen to have drawn an example from those events. One closes one's eyes to the fact that the holocaust was a program of mass murder of millions of private citizens, conceived and implemented by the government. It was a unique program without historical parallel with respect to decision making, planning, and ruthless implementation, utilizing all the available technological resources, often at the expense of the war effort. Even Stalin's purges and horrible mass murders pale in comparison with the holocaust. The example of the mass eradication of the Armenians by the Turks might come closer, but even this was basically a local and ancient ethnic conflict. In contrast, the Nazis carried on a prolonged extermination of people whose only common denominator was that they belonged to, had belonged to, or were descendants of people belonging to a certain religion.

Vrba spoke with the same intense but nevertheless distanced and occasionally slightly ironic voice as in Lanzmann's film. I looked around. We were sitting in a first-class Parisian restaurant, surrounded by elegant people, having a very nice dinner in the best French tradition. The street was still filled with people strolling casually by, enjoying the fine, warm fall evening. We were again immersed in the dark and unbearable subject. But which is the true reality? Who is fooling himself?

No one. Reality is an optical illusion, like the work by Escher in which black birds fly toward the right, and white birds toward the left. It is not possible to see both at the same time. They mutually exclude one another. Most people prefer to look at the white birds. They may be aware of the black birds, at least at an intellectual level, but emotionally they try to exclude them. A similar psychological mechanism must have been in operation in the concentration camps. In his essay "Individual and Mass Behavior in Extreme Situations," Bruno Bettelheim describes how the prisoners tried to "exteriorize" their situation.[10] Their attitude might be described in the following terms: What is happening cannot possibly happen to me. Therefore it is not real. I must be able to separate myself as subject from myself as object. I must protect myself, my attitudes, and my values so that I can remain the same person in the unlikely event that I manage to survive this.

The wish to concentrate on the white birds even under objectively completely black circumstances may reflect a survival mechanism. Relatives of those who had already been deported and who realized that they were to be the next targets, as well as similarly deceived people elsewhere in the same country or in other lands, resorted to similar mechanisms of selective understanding. It is hardly surprising that neither they nor the even more distant large masses that were not affected by the atrocities chose to disbelieve all rumors about mass murder. They preferred to write them off as heinous propaganda, pure fabrication.

But why did the three of us, with Jacob listening, choose to spend that beautiful Saturday in Paris compulsively focusing our attention on the black birds? We were all citizens of free countries, living well in peaceful times. Were we haunted by feelings of guilt toward the dead? Were we afraid that the whole experience would recur if we let go? We knew that the wide and relentless river of history is rarely influenced by knowledge of the past. In no more than one or two generations, archives of extreme horror turn into scraps of faded paper, with no more influence than dried leaves. I suddenly felt that we were like a traveler with a fear of flying, forcing himself to stay awake and keep his seatbelt buckled during the entire flight, obsessed with the idea that the plane would surely crash if he were to fall asleep. But perhaps we had other motives. Perhaps we wanted to feel a solidarity with each other by selecting a more or less taboo subject for our conversation, one avoided by most others. Or did we try to perform a kind of autopsy, using our brains to understand what human minds are capable of at their worst? Have we appointed our brains to serve as the pathologist and the cadaver at the same time?

I was suddenly overcome by an irresistible urge to change the subject. I asked Jacob if he remembered the time some years earlier when he had asked me to present a lecture at the Collège de France. Following an ancient tradition, we entered the small faculty lounge prior to the lecture, where we happened to run into writer, philosopher, and political scientist Raymond Aron. He mentioned to Jacob that Robert Schuman, the former finance minister in De Gaulle's administration, had just published his autobiography describing, among other things, his wartime experiences. He praised Jacob's achievements as a soldier in De Gaulle's army in Africa. Apparently Jacob had refused to abandon a badly wounded comrade and carried him a vast distance, at great risk to his own life.

I had heard previously that Jacob was one of De Gaulle's most decorated soldiers, but I had never heard of that episode. Jacob seemed embarrassed, and he didn't want to discuss it further. He asked instead what Schuman's book was like. Not particularly good, Aron replied. Schuman is incapable of discussing anguish (*l'angoisse*). Who could discuss l'angoisse? "Andre Malraux," Jacob and Aron said almost simultaneously.

This episode occurred more than two decades before our visit to Paris. And now Jacob has written about anguish himself. Suddenly, all three of us begin talking about his book, using different words but all exhibiting much appreciation. Jacob listened, looked away, remained silent. His description of anguish seizes the reader, even though it does not necessarily refer to events of the battlefield. His description of an episiode in which he passed only yards from the muzzle of a German soldier's rifle conveys no fear. Inexplicably, the soldier did not fire. Anxiety came at the moment of long-desired victory, after Jacob had been seriously wounded during the Allied drive toward Paris. He was severely disabled and hospitalized for an extended period of time, abandoned by his friends and with a few close relatives as his only human contacts.

His less courageous friends, who had chosen to remain in occupied France, had already completed much of their medical education. Jacob had barely begun his. The girl whom he loved had become engaged to someone else, and his hopes of becoming a surgeon lay in ruins. I have often heard biologists say that there are many excellent surgeons, and that it was really quite fortunate that the cruelty of fate prevented Jacob from becoming a physician. But anyone who makes such a thoughtless remark cannot have tried very hard to imagine how difficult it was for Jacob: the bitterness at finding himself left out of everything and separated from everyone; his disabilities, the excruciating pain with every step; the cold room, the lonely environment that seemed to be his obvious fate. The feeling of being the least clever of his entire school class, even of his whole generation. The thought of enormous potential gone to waste, of times gone by without any accomplishments. The potential of life being utilized to the full by everyone but him. The brief meeting with his old love, real but still unreal, faded like old photographs turned yellow in the album. The camaraderie of the war years, now an unreal memory. The impossibility, the unwillingness, the inability to say "we" in any context. An abhorrence of all political parties and their self-serving propaganda. The search for the murderer and his victims in strange faces. The blurring of the borderline between those who fought against the Nazis and those who profited from them. Five years of terrible tragedy had vanished suddenly, they had submerged like stones under the sea while the world continued as if nothing had happened.

The relentless flow of our accounts of what we had read left Jacob apparently unmoved. He didn't say a word. From my previous conversations and correspondence with him, I knew that he would readily respond to questions related to science and practical issues, but he was unwilling to comment on the reactions of others to his nonscientific writings.

In the middle of this conversation between three who had read a book written by the silent fourth, Vrba suddenly said, "But there is one detail in the book that has given me a sleepless night."

We were all flabbergasted. How could anything in Jacob's book upset Vrba? We knew that Vrba's own book is the safest drug against sleep. Vrba, the man who had experienced the ultimate hell himself, a hell that is difficult to even try to describe in any human language? In comparison, Jacob's book is filled with simple tales and charming little stories. Could we have missed something?

The episode that had upset Vrba dealt with the first lecture Jacob had to give in English to the international audience of scientists at the Pasteur Institute. He felt very insecure and decided to read his talk from the manuscript with his strong French accent. His friend and colleague Jean Weiglé, a well-known scientist who could, in Jacob's view, discern subtle signs not visible to others, advised him strongly against reading from his manuscript. "Your talk will be much better if you speak freely, despite your imperfect English," he said.

But Jacob absolutely refused to listen. Just before he was to step up to the podium, however, Jacob noticed with panic that his manuscript had vanished. There was nothing he could do! Filled with fear, he walked up to the podium and presented his talk in halting but quite comprehensible English. It had obviously gone well. Weiglé told him after the lecture that he had stolen the manuscript. "It was the best way to convince you that you should never read a talk from a paper. You did beautifully," was his congratulatory comment.

"How can a scientist do something like that to a young colleague?" Vrba exclaimed, red with anger. "I would never have believed that of someone like Weiglé!"

I had a vague sense of déjà vu. I remembered George Orwell's *Nineteen Eighty-Four*. In his nightmarish view of the Stalinist future, the Thought Police tortures its political prisoners in the Ministry of Love, a large pyramidal and windowless building containing all kinds of unimaginably hellish instruments. But the worst tortures were carried out in Room 101, a plain room lacking any special equipment. In this room each prisoner was confronted with what he feared the most. Orwell's hero had to endure the threat of ferocious rats gnawing at his face. But what is it that Vrba, the man Elie Wiesel called "an authentic hero," could find in

Room 101 instead of rats? Why was he so shaken by Weiglé's little practical joke, a prank that Jacob himself admitted turned out to be so helpful in the long run?

It was a criminal thing to do, regardless of the result. It was theft, Vrba repeated, still visibly upset. A good scientist should not be allowed to commit such a reprehensible act, because the search for scientific truth makes certain ethical demands on those who practice science. Vrba's position was consistent with the argument he had made earlier in the afternoon, when he asserted that German scientists who utilized material from the concentration camps and, in the worst cases, even participated in the executions, were charlatans. They could not be called scientists. But Weiglé was a highly respected scientist.

"No, it's not that simple, unfortunately," Benno replied. Vrba's criteria could be met only if the basic definition of science were changed to include ethical precepts, especially the principle of righteousness. The traditional concept of science, however, makes no allowance for any such reformulation. How do we judge an ordinary person who in most situations behaves in accordance with accepted moral norms, but who does not hesitate to steal when there is no risk of being caught? Think of all the plundering and looting that has taken place even in the most civilized of countries during so many wars, earthquakes, floods, and other disasters. Is a scientist who steals results from other scientists and uses them in his own research necessarily a bad scientist? Possibly yes and possibly no, depending on the quality of the work to which he applies the stolen material. In most cases it is only the victim who cares that he has been robbed. It is generally very difficult for others to take positions in instances of alleged "idea stealing" in the scientific world, to follow all the claims and counter-claims that are usually so trivial that they arouse no more than a yawn when the victim prattles on about it. Ideas are regarded as common property, and it is usually very difficult to know where and when an idea first arose. Some are born from the Zeitgeist, occasionally in several places simultaneously. The originator might be as anonymous as the first author of a ballad or a common popular joke.

"And how," Benno continued, "are we to judge those who would not hesitate to commit atrocities in the name of a current reigning ideology, during wars, revolutions, totalitarian dictatorships, when the killing of undesirables and persecuted minorities is a state-sanctioned duty?" Scientists need not necessarily participate, as Mengele did, in the atrocities, but they can be easily tempted to forget about moral considerations when their scientific interests take priority. One of the most prominent figures in German neuropathology, Professor Hallervorden, said to an SS doctor, "Since you are killing all these people anyhow, you might just as well send me their brains." By the end of the war, he had received 697 brains from murdered psychiatric patients. He knew exactly what he wanted and why. He was not trying to identify specific changes in the brains of psychiatric patients, because he already knew that no such changes could be detected with the methods available at the time. He remained within the realm of what was possible, and thereby made contributions that were significant and remain a firm part of current neuropathology.Hallervorden retained his professorship after the war. Many scientific papers and doctoral theses have been based on material he collected. Reports of the executions are still to be found in the archives of the institutions, written neatly by the "euthanasia doctor" or by the SS doctor, indicating with pride the precise time when the brain was fixed: "Two hours after death," "completely fresh," and so on.

When Hallervorden died in 1965, many laudatory obituaries were written. His colleague Prof. Spatz eulogized him as a great scientist and a deeply moral man.[11] He was described as a devoted follower of the ethical philosophy of Kant. This is exemplified by his absolute focus on scientific problems, his sense of duty, and his support of young research colleagues. According to these descriptions, he was a modest man, completely different from the autocratic *Geheimrat* type.

During relatively peaceful times, when professors have a stable and reasonable income, it is difficult to imagine that scientists can act criminally, steal, rob, and even murder, Benno continued. We cannot conceive that there might be a connection between their world and that of Mengele. But we cannot escape that easily. Mengele's most immediate supervisor, Professor Ottmar Baron von Verschuer, expressed his great appreciation for Mengele's "splendid utilization of the enormous potential of Auschwitz for scientific research." He was himself one of the leading "race biologists" and Mengele's closest scientific mentor. He also died an honored man, many years after the end of the war.[12]

The most detailed and thorough description of Mengele's horrible activities in Auschwitz can be found in a book written shortly after the war by his closest professional assistant, the Hungarian Jewish pathologist Miklós Nyiszli. He himself was a prisoner under constant threat of death, like all Jews at Auschwitz, and he was a member of the so-called *Sonderkommando,* who were murdered and replaced at regular intervals. Nyiszli survived, thanks to his skill and knowledge, which Mengele took advantage of. He had a well-equipped pathology laboratory at his disposal, situated no more than sixty yards from the gas chambers. It takes very strong nerves to read his book.[13] In his foreword, Bruno Bettelheim says, "It is an unbelievable story, but we all know it is true. We wish to forget it. It just does not fit into our current system of thoughts. And rather than to reshape them, we wish to dismiss the story of the German extermination camps. If we could, we would prefer to think it never happened. Since this is impossible, we prefer to forget about it so that we need not come to terms with its nightmarish perspectives." Bettelheim characterizes the attitude of the doctors and of the general community as a kind of inertia, a tendency to consider even the most heinous atrocities "business as usual."

He continues: "All this would be past history except that the very same 'business as usual' makes us forget two things: that twentieth century men like us sent millions into the gas chambers and that millions of men like us walked to death without resistance. . . . In the deepest sense, the walk to the gas chamber was only the last consequence of the philosophy of 'business as usual.'"

Bettelheim also points to the great danger that stems from our respect for technical competence. In this regard, he is in full agreement with Benno when he says, "Auschwitz is gone, but as long as this attitude remains with us we cannot be protected from criminal indifference to life at its core."

Nyiszli calls Mengele a "criminal doctor" and the greatest felon in the history of the world. But at the same time he is filled with admiration for what he considers Mengele's scientific interest, his persistent, focused work, his talent for observation, his precision. Mengele passed out innumerable death sentences and even murdered with his own hands. His monstrosities are perfectly apparent. But what about the German doctors who competed for the empty spaces in the psychiatric hospitals after the completion of the euthanasia programs there, or of the other intellectuals so eager to assume the positions vacated by the Jewish professors? Their private ambitions could be easily hidden behind a facade of altruism. The hospital rooms should be emptied to reduce the costs of medical care. The program to extinguish *lebensunwertes Leben* (lives not worthy to be lived), as in the case of the execution of chronically ill patients or mentally retarded infants, could be disguised as a humanitarian activity. The absurd concepts of the race biologists could easily be justified in a political climate in which it was generally accepted that the hereditary factors of the nation should be purged of "Jewish genes," condemned by the Führer as the "cancer" of the nation.

From this point, the road led straight to mass murder, euphemistically called "the final solution." The lies grew along with the murders, like twins. The criminal leadership divided the job behind this smokescreen: Himmler's main task was to kill, Göring's job was to steal valuables and property, and Goebbels was responsible for all the official lying. Hitler amalgamated all three of these aims within himself. Why should science be an exception in a state ruled by this triumvirate of murderers, thieves, and liars?

"Here is where we differ," Benno said, turning to Vrba. "Science is incompatible with lying and secrecy about scientific data, but there is no ethical prohibition against robbery and murder in a society in which such actions are sanctioned. Murder is not legitimized in our time and culture, and we have difficulties in understanding the experience of the Nazi era. It tells us that not even the worst crime a human being can commit against another is deterrent in itself, if sanctioned by the political leadership."

Vrba was not convinced by Benno's argument. He persisted in his belief that scientists who participate in murder cannot be considered true scientists. At best, they might be considered "well-groomed curs" (*frisierte Schnauzen*), polished and well-camouflaged opportunists.

Toward the end of the evening, it became obvious that Benno and Vrba had become friends despite their differences of opinion. They agreed to disagree. But Benno and I wondered why Vrba had to cling to the image of the righteous scientist? Why would scientists differ from others? Was Vrba grasping at straws to save his faith in humanity? In that case, what right do we have to take that from him?

Where is my remaining horror, my own personal Room 101? In his last book, *The Drowned and the Saved,* Primo Levi wrote,

Above and beyond our personal experiences, we have collectively witnessed a fundamental, unexpected event, fundamental precisely because unexpected, not foreseen by anyone. It took place in the teeth of all forecasts; it happened in Europe; incredibly, it happened that an entire civilized people, just issued from the fervid cultural flowering of Weimar, followed a buffoon whose figure today inspires laughter, and yet Adolf Hitler was obeyed and his praises were sung right up to the catastrophe. It happened, therefore it can happen again: this is the core of what we have to say. . . . It is not very probable that all factors that unleashed the Nazi madness will again occur simultaneously but precursory signs loom before us. Violence, "useful" or "useless," is there before our eyes: it snakes either through sporadic and private episodes, or government lawlessness, both in what we call the first and the second worlds, that is to say, the parliamentary democracies and countries in the Communist bloc. In the third world it is endemic or epidemic. It only awaits its new buffoon (there is no dearth of candidates) to organize it, legalize it, declare it necessary and mandatory, and so contaminate the world. Few countries can be considered immune to a future tide of violence generated by intolerance, lust for power, economic difficulties, religious or political fanaticism, and racialist attritions. It is therefore necessary to sharpen our senses, distrust the prophets, the enchanters, those who speak and write "beautiful words" unsupported by intelligent reasons.

Is that my Room 101, the fear of oblivion, the fear that it can all happen again if we are not constantly reminded of the past? Possibly so. But I know that there is yet another room, the innermost and most terrible of all.

In the fall of 1988, Benno Müller-Hill organized a conference in Cologne. In contrast to most scientific conferences in which a particular theme or set of themes is chosen, Müller-Hill's symposium had the broad title "Medical Science without Compassion." The meeting was opened by Vrba and Hermann Langbein, also a survivor of Auschwitz and an unpretentious yet incisive witness of the horrors of that hellish planet. After them came a number of experts on the ideological history of Nazism and the principles of its murderous doctors and scientists. We also heard descriptions of the equally horrendous experiments that the Japanese carried out in one of their gigantic, specially constructed camps in Manchuria—an appalling fact that is still hushed-up in modern Japan.

But unethical experimentation was not limited to the totalitarian states. It was for me quite a shocking revelation to hear about the deceptive experiments sponsored by the CIA on volunteers during the McCarthy era in the United States. Those were times when parts of the American government were obsessed with fear of Stalinist "brainwashing" and spent large sums of money on "behavior-modulation experiments" with LSD and other mind-altering drugs. Hidden cameras and observation stations were part of the armamentarium. In the end, these experiments did not result in the "elimination" of the test subjects, but it was particularly troublesome that the studies were carried out with support from a federal body, in the world's largest democracy, in peacetime.

As I sat in the meeting, trying to formulate some concluding remarks as I had been asked to do, I detected a recurrent underlying theme in most of the talks. Not even the worst crimes that were discussed at the meeting had been committed by psychopaths, sadists, or the kind of monsters that the mass media and crime films like so much to portray for impressionable young people. Some of the leaders, like Hitler—in a class by himself—and possibly also the bloodhound-like Senator McCarthy, were undoubtedly psychopaths. But this convenient label cannot be applied to most of the functionaries. On the contrary, they were conformists and good citizens whose activities had been sanctioned by the system and whose consciences were "clean." After all, they were performing "patriotic work" and were being rewarded with good incomes and promotions.

The real problem is the *conformity* itself, not the atrocities and the inhumanities per se. According to American historians who have studied the experiments in Manchuria, the Japanese treated their prisoners very well during the First World War. However, less than three decades later, they treated prisoners with exceptional cruelty. Many of us remember the film *The Bridge on the River*

Kwai, if nothing else. Our Chinese, Korean, and other East Asian friends have much to add to that story. What had happened to that polite and friendly nation between the two world wars to explain such an enormous change?

Historians attribute this national transformation to changes in Japanese leaders and their ideology. During the First World War, after two centuries of isolation, Japanese politicians were intent on contacts and openness toward the West. They even considered the prisoners of war to be human beings through whom they wished to foster contacts with the West. During the Second World War the country was led by the military, which wanted to revive the traditional spirit of war. A Japanese soldier was never to surrender to the enemy—to do so was regarded as the most cowardly act of all. His duty was to commit suicide. The same judgment was applied to English and American prisoners of war. Those who surrendered deserved no respect as human beings. Is it possible that the attitudes of a whole group or an entire nation can be changed so easily by one or a small number of leaders? Apparently so, especially if loyalty to the leaders or the system is more important than one's own conscience.

I looked around the lecture hall in Cologne. We all agreed in our condemnation of unethical and criminal experiments with human beings. But the doctors and the "scientists" who performed the experiments were merely products of their time and of the society that had sanctioned their activities. Even the general population had quietly accepted, tolerated, or in any case ignored what they were doing.

We also are children of our own time. In this time and in this society, it is correct and praiseworthy to condemn cruelty and murder, to regard those who practice them as criminals. We feel righteous in our indignation, and we are fully convinced that we would be incapable of doing such things. But are we not also conformists within the spirit of our own times? Can we be sure that we would have behaved differently if we had lived in that time and place? Don't we have to prove first that we can go against the stream, follow our own consciences, even if it may involve economic hardships or injure our careers, even if we are condemned by those closest to us, and even if it leads, in the extreme case, to ultimate punishment? How can our moral indignation be considered reliable in the absence of such proof?

The gap between us and the era of Hitler is fortunately so great that the whole question seems absurd. But the CIA-supported experiments that were carried out in a free society awakens a far greater and more imminent fear.

At the time of the conference in Cologne I had just finished a very difficult but necessary project. As so often in the past, I had to prepare a large research grant application, the worst kind of work I know. I have to write down what I already know and have already published. I learn nothing new from it. It has to be written clearly and concisely to be competitive. It must contain detailed plans for the future, even though both I and the funding agency realize that such plans are purely fictitious. In reality, the scientific problem has to be pursued step by step, without the constraints of a rigidly determined plan. This is the only part of my work that I dislike. For a period of two or three months I feel as if I am in prison. All my energy and the pleasure of work is gone, but I have to finish it! It is like climbing a high mountain.

Imagine if someone were to offer me a grant, enough for my entire department to function, in exchange for some experiments that might not take more than a fraction of my time and could be done with the left hand, or even one finger. This is just how the CIA agents went about it when they persuaded the American sociologists to carry out their unethical LSD experiments.

Would I have the courage and strength to say no to experiments that I consider unethical? I hope and believe that I would, but only a self-deceiving hypocrite would claim that he knows this for certain, before he could prove it to be true.

Can I be 100 percent certain that I would say no?

This recurrent thought is my Room 101.

6

The Fatherless

For as long as I can remember, I have known that my father was not alive. He died when I was one year old. I have heard a lot about him and have seen many pictures of him. He is looking at me even now as I write this. Father, little brother, stranger—you could have been my son by now. What kind of person were you, what did your voice sound like, what did you dream about? You hide behind the veil of the family legend that describes how hard you worked and how you encouraged others to use their own initiative. Were you really like that?

I have only one object that you left behind, a well-worn old book from the turn of the century, filled with your dated, pencilled notations in the margins. The book is a collection of short stories by a rather mediocre Hungarian author. You were reading it on the train, on the way to your army unit that was mobilized during the First World War. Did you jot down your thoughts in the margins of the book because you did not have any other paper, or were you inspired by what you were reading? You were only twenty-nine years old, but you did not believe that you were to become much older. You were filled with anxiety and were convinced that you would never see your home again, but you had no desire to die. I cannot find the slightest trace of patriotic zeal in your notes, nothing like the feelings that are said to have filled most other recruits during the early stages of the war. On the contrary, you were full of bitter feelings toward those "villains" who governed the world and brought ruin upon all.

Harsh, indignant letters written with a quivering pencil. Was the train shaking too much? Your anguish seizes and agitates—it pervades this son whom you were to beget eight years later. He who is old enough now to be your father is looking at your face and writing about you in a language that you didn't understand.

You didn't know then what your son knows now—that you were to survive the war, marry my mother, and start a prosperous business. You did not know that you were to leave your grieving wife and baby son, your parents and brothers, less than ten years after that train ride, after they had all been forced to watch your long and painful battle against a bacterium with the springlike name *Streptococcus viridans*, which had infected your heart valves and which today would be quickly eradicated with some penicillin. Even less could you suspect then that your early death would allow you to escape something far worse. You were spared from sharing the horrible fate of your mother and brothers, the ultimate form of human degradation: death in the gas chambers of Auschwitz. Through your death you rescued my mother and me, for after you died we moved from your village to Budapest, where my mother's parents and brothers lived and where a series of coincidences saved us from Auschwitz.

Father, little brother, my unknown young friend and my creator, how lucky you were never to learn how reality could become so much more brutal than you could ever have imagined during that train ride. Not even in your worst anguish would you have suspected how justified you were in your abhorrence of those villains who govern the world.

Stranger, I have often longed for you. At times I have missed you so much that I would gladly have given my life just for one chance to talk with you. Only much later did I start to realize that it is precisely because of your absence that I have become what I am now. Jean-Paul Sartre's biography, *Les Mots*, made me aware for the first time of the unique psychological characteristics of the fatherless child. I could readily identify with some of the traits he describes. Sartre writes,

There is no good father, that's the rule. Don't lay the blame on men but on the bond of paternity, which is rotten. To beget children, nothing better; to *have* them, what iniquity! Had my father lived, he would have lain on me at full length and would have crushed me. As luck had it, he died young. Amidst Aeneas and his fellows who carry their Anchises on their backs, I move from shore to shore, alone and hating those invisible begetters who bestraddle their sons all their life long. I left behind me a young man who did not have time to be my father and who could now be my son. Was it a good thing or a bad? I don't know. But I readily subscribe to the verdict of an eminent psychologist: I have no Superego. . . . .That accounts, beyond a doubt, for my incredible levity (*mon incroyable légèreté*). I am not a leader, nor do I aspire to become one. Command, obey, it's all one. The bossiest of men commands in the name of another—his father—and transmits the abstract acts of violence which he puts up with. Never in my life have I given an order without laughing, without making others laugh. It is because I am not consumed by the canker of power: I was not taught obedience.[1]

Yes, in some ways I readily recognized these traits in myself: the lack of respect for the mighty, for all hierarchical and patriarchal systems; the tendency, the self-assurance or, if you like, the impertinence of attempting to judge all situations on my own instead of looking for guidance and direction from others; the courage to make decisions quickly without necessarily asking how others would customarily react in a similar situation; the inability to understand that others may function in completely different ways until I get a richly deserved punch in the nose or slap on the wrist.

Arrogance? Yes, you can certainly call it that, but an arrogance combined with humility stemming from my own *incroyable légèreté* of the fatherless. Too much self-assurance? Yes, sometimes. Decisive and problem-solving determination? Yes, perhaps that too. The searchlight that darts through my selective autobiographical memory picks out the decision to go to Sweden only a few seconds after I was asked if I wanted to go. There is the additional example of my escape, on a moment's impulse, from the deportation train at the railway station—a decision that had high survival value, as it turned out, but also carried great risks. The daring choice of devoting myself to a purely scientific career in Sweden, in spite of the virtual absence of any possibilities for advancement in my chosen field; the risks of declining a number of attractive job offers in the United States; the courage or foolhardiness to venture into unexplored scientific fields, to place my complete trust in unfamiliar people; my decision to marry a woman I had known for only eight days. To this day, my inner self-critic is brave or arrogant enough to characterize these decisions as positive.

Have I made many foolish decisions in the same way? Yes, many. They are largely erased or hidden in a special chamber, protected from inspection. But along the way that leads to this chamber of horrors there are a number of relatively trivial episodes, not sufficiently dangerous to be erased or locked away, not sufficiently important to be emphasized. Am I proud of them, do I feel ashamed of them?

Both, I would say. I am proud of some, ashamed of others, and there are a few of which I am both proud and ashamed at the same time. They include two instances in which I impulsively acted as a strikebreaker. By the usual Swedish standards I should be ashamed of these actions, but I can see only their positive sides.

The first instance occurred in Budapest in 1945 when I broke a students' strike. The communist-infiltrated student organization had ordered all students to boycott registration at the university to protest a minimal but additional fee. I smelled a rat, although I was unaware that a power struggle was in progress between a small but very active communist group (which took over the student organization the following year) and several groups of more moderate but less vociferous students.

I was absolutely furious. Once again somebody wanted to prevent me from studying. Wasn't the official restricted quota for admission of Jewish students during the fascist period bad enough? Was it really possible that my own student organization would now stop me? I realized that one must be loyal to fellow students. Besides, veiled threats had been made against anyone who might dare to defy what was described as "practically 100 percent voluntary support" of the strike.

I was standing in a large and densely packed crowd of students in front of the registration office. No one moved. The strike leaders were holding up their posters while the registrars sat impassive behind their counters.

I glanced at the strike leaders. I had no respect for them whatsoever. I didn't fully understand their motives, but I suspected that they had reasons for their actions other than solidarity with the plight of poor students.

Suddenly I was overwhelmed with rage. Could my fellow students now accomplish what both the Hungarian and German fascists had earlier failed to achieve—to prevent me from studying?

Resolutely I approached the registration counter. The strike leaders ordered me to turn back and one of them even threatened to bring in the police to stop me. I never found out whether this was a bit of wishful thinking on their part, or if they anticipated what was to come with the communist takeover the following year. But their shouts increased my resolve and my confidence that I was doing the right thing. I went ahead.

At the counter I asked the clerk to register me. When he finished, I turned around and found myself facing a dozen furious strike leaders and a large group of silent students. They didn't make a sound—no whistling or hooting at me. Suddenly several other students broke off from the crowd and walked up to the counter to register. Then two more, then three, then ten followed. After fifteen minutes the strike was over. I had no feeling of any victory, only a great relief over the prospect of starting my studies soon and indifference to any political repercussions.

I remembered that incident some years later, after I had become a young professor, a father of three children, and the proud owner of a newly purchased house, thanks to a loan from the Swedish Physicians Union. One day I received an announcement from the union that all of its members would be required to join the physicians strike then in progress, including professors and scientists who never saw patients.

I was seized by the same rage that I had felt several decades earlier in Budapest. Is there anybody who can prevent me from going to my laboratory? Was the union going to keep me from my work? Shall I follow the orders of an organization that had wanted to keep out all foreign medical students like myself, and gave in only after strong political pressures, due to the shortage of doctors? First and foremost, I had to be faithful to myself, to my collaborators, and to my work. I wrote a letter protesting the forced participation of nonclinical members in the strike, and I requested that they excuse us from this obligation. I got a speedy reply. Their demand was irrevocable. If I persisted, the loan for my house would be cancelled.

I resigned from the union, had my loan cancelled, and managed by other means. I felt wonderful.

I have never regretted my actions during those two strikes, although some may think that I acted in an asocial way. But I can recall other impulsive actions that were more problematic for me. I remember two of these episodes in particular.

During the winter of 1961, after one of the most difficult personal crises in my life, Eva and I decided to take a skiing vacation in Switzerland. Two of our children, Peter, who was then eight years old, and Margareta, then six, came with us. We were booked in tourist class on Swissair, and we started our journey dressed in our ski outfits. The plane made an intermediate stop in Düsseldorf. At the entrance to the transit hall, the names of all passengers were checked against the manifest, as had to be done before the computer age. Our names were not on the list. I showed our tickets, Stockholm to Zürich, all O.K. The stewardess called the airline office and told us that their people in Stockholm had apparently forgotten to include our names on the passenger list, and the Düsseldorf office had therefore already sold our seats. I told her that we had to get to our destination, that we were expected that night and had only one week for our vacation. I asked when we would be able to continue our flight. Not until tomorrow, was the answer. No, that is simply impossible, I said. Sleepless nights and the whole nightmarish cycle of sedatives and stimulants that I had been on during the previous few weeks had gotten my adrenaline flowing. I demanded to talk to her supervisor.

The supervisor came, a smartly uniformed man. His firm and austerely pompous German style reminded me of Nazi officers during the Second World War. I explained the situation to him in a somewhat irritated tone and added that under no circumstances could we imagine spending the night in Düsseldorf. He turned his back to me and ordered the stewardess to "Go take the gentleman's hand luggage off the plane." Then he turned around sharply and left.

Suddenly I was furious. I grabbed my children's hands resolutely and marched with them toward the door marked *Ausgang verboten* that led directly out to the tarmac. Eva pleaded desperately with me to stop, but in vain. I threw the door open and dragged the children out with me while the airport personnel were shouting warnings— *"verboten!"* and *"zurück!"* I continued on toward the plane, which at the time was being refueled. Again the airline personnel tried to stop me, but I shoved them aside, not violently but firmly. More shouts of *"verboten!"* were now mixed with *"Sind Sie verrückt?"* I pushed the steward and air hostesses aside, went up the stairway, entered the plane, and sat down implacably in the first seat I could find. The captain appeared and ordered me to leave the plane immediately. I answered that he would have to call the police—I had no intention of leaving voluntarily. Following a quick consultation between the airport personnel and the flight crew outside the plane, they all returned, but amazingly, their behavior had changed completely. They were now extremely polite. *Of course* it had all been a mistake, and *naturally* they could arrange for us to fly to Zürich on the same flight if we were willing to move to two seats in the first-class section and have the children sit on our laps. But first we had to promise not to sue the airline.

My first impulse was to say something nasty about some of my earlier experiences in which I had seen those ramrod German backs forced to bend suddenly. But I managed to control my urge. I promised, and our flight continued.

I suspect that there is a connection between my behavior in this dubious incident and the absence of a father. In spite of the successful outcome of that confrontation, I was painfully aware that I should not have dragged the children with me.

I acted even worse once in the 1960s, after I had returned from a trip to Moscow. The journey had been both edifying and depressing. Some of the contrasts bordered on the surreal. I experienced the warm friendship of my Russian colleagues, but also the utter impossibility of their personal and scientific problems. The genuine enthusiasm and obvious education of the concert public contrasted with the drab hopelessness and endless frustration of everyday life, awakening in me not only feelings of sympathy and irritation but also a deep sense of guilt for feeling irritated. It was as if I were banging my head against the wall. The haughtily hostile "apparatus" did its best to block the way wherever you looked. The almighty Government and its uniformed or plainclothes agents took on a great sense of self-importance; individuals were slaves whose right to exist was directly proportional to their willingness and ability to serve the state and to follow its often meaningless whims without any ideas of their own.

It was as if our Swedish Jante law[2] had been taken to its ultimate and most absurd conclusion.

After a thousand complications, I finally arrived at Stockholm's Arlanda airport. I took a deep breath, relieved and happy—my fatigue had completely vanished. The beautiful Swedish summer had reached its peak, and I wanted to go for a swim before plunging into the accumulated work at home.

I followed the signs to the Arlanda beach and found a pleasant spot in an enclosed area with clearly demarcated boundaries, even in the water. There were many children playing. I jumped into the water and began swimming out into the bay. Suddenly I heard a voice on a loudspeaker ordering me to "turn back at once!" I became furious. Isn't there a law in Sweden that guarantees the right of everybody to use any of the waters? Don't I have the right to swim wherever I want in my own country? Did I go from the ashes into the fire? I ignored the call and continued swimming.

Within a few minutes a motorboat was speeding toward me, with two infuriated lifeguards on board.

"Turn back immediately!" The command sounded just like an order in Moscow.

"What authority do you have to order me to turn around?"

"We are in charge here on this beach."

"Is there a law that says I can't swim here? Isn't the water here free for all?"

"You are not allowed to swim here!"

"What law says I can't swim here?"

"You are setting a very poor example for the children."

"I agree, you are absolutely right, and I do apologize. But is there any law that prohibits me from swimming here?"

They were speechless.

"OK, go and get the police. I'll just have to take the consequences for what I have done."

I turned and continued swimming out into the bay. The guards returned to shore and no police ever came.

I wasn't particularly proud of my behavior. I realized that I had acted improperly, but I also knew that I would never have done so had it not been for the combination of my exhaustion and my experiences in Moscow. Am I making excuses for myself? Perhaps. What does the absence of an authoritative father figure have to do with it ? Possibly nothing, possibly a great deal. Would I like to live in a society in which everyone behaved like that? No, never. Was Sartre wrong to condemn Aeneas for carrying his father Anchises on his back? Did he get himself into the same kind of senselessly stubborn situation, allowing his existentialist freedom of choice to get out of control when in his old age he distributed Maoist leaflets on the streets of Paris—just as the bloody cultural revolution in China was taking place and not very long before the start of the horrible ideological massacres in Kampuchea?

When the Hungarian head of state, János Kádár, came to Sweden on an official visit in the spring of 1987, Prime Minister Ingvar Carlsson hosted a dinner party at the foreign ministry in his honor. Swedish politicians, academicians, and businessmen were invited to the dinner, together with many members of the Swedish-Hungarian colony. Only a few years earlier the Swedish-Hungarians would have declined the invitation, but now most of them showed up. After the revolution in Hungary in 1956, Kádár was seen as a traitor. Years earlier, during the Stalin epoch, he had been imprisoned in Rákosis jail, but he was released during the time of the official repudiation of Stalin. In 1956 he became a member of Imre Nagy's revolutionary government—a regime that later came to be denounced as counterrevolutionary. Kádár was the one who asked the Russians to intervene against his own government, and it was with their help that he came to power.

But after several years of condemnation from all over the world, the harsh criticism of Kádár began to subside, and eventually it gave way to a growing sense of amazement and, at times, admiration. Alone among the Eastern bloc leaders—and two decades before Gorbachev—Kádár had secretly changed the system from top to bottom, totally from within, gradually, consistently, and along progressive lines. At first most people thought that the changes were only cosmetic, mere nuances in the Communist power structure. Kádár changed one of the main tenets of the official state paranoia, the fundamentally Stalinist concept of "He who is not with us is against us," to "He who is not against us is with us." People started talking about "socialism with a human face." Freedom of speech increased, slowly at first but then with increasing speed. Some subjects, such as sensitive questions about the presence of Soviet troops in the country, the acts of the secret police, or private contacts with Israel, remained taboo. But eventually the secret police was dissolved and diplomatic relations with Israel were established. But the existence of Soviet troops continued to be a particularly sensitive issue. (They were withdrawn only after the recent downfall of the communist regime.) The Hungarian people were increasingly free to travel, and the harsh restrictions against foreign books and newspapers disappeared. The private sector, originally forbidden and later quietly tolerated, was now "out in full bloom."

Even occasional visitors could notice the considerable differences between the happy and colorful Hungary and her gloomier Eastern bloc neighbors. In the cabarets of Budapest comedians ridiculed the government and its deficiencies, the corrupt and incompetent party officials, but they never joked about the Soviets. As the mistakes of the Hungarian leaders came to be discussed more frequently and more openly, demands for reform became stronger. A steady stream of literary works, whose publication would previously have been unthinkable, began to appear, severely critical of the role of the party during the Stalin period. The subsequent avalanche, as we now see it in retrospect, was a direct continuation of this process. "The counterrevolution" of 1956 has been reconsidered, Imre Nagy and his government have been rehabilitated, the period between 1953 and 1956 and the role of the communists has been totally reevaluated. Kádár had passed away before the ultimate downfall of the communist regime; embittered, sick, and old, having been blamed for the economic crisis of his administration and for his own fate as well as the tragic fate of his friends. But no one can erase the pioneering role that Kádár played as the first East European communist leader to liberate and reform the system. His own downfall can be looked upon as a consequence of the process he started himself.

At the time of the foreign ministry dinner in Stockholm, these events were still in the future. Kádár was still the supreme leader in Hungary, and Gorbachev's liberalization in the USSR was in its early stages. It was, therefore, quite a sensation that Kádár was the first East bloc politician to raise the subject of Raoul Wallenberg during the speech at the dinner with Ingvar Carlsson, even though Kádár described Wallenberg as an example of good Swedish-Hungarian relations. He mentioned only that Wallenberg had rescued thousands of people from the Nazi persecutions, but never said that most of the victims were Jews. He also avoided saying anything about Wallenberg's fate, but the fact that he dealt with the matter at all was a major step forward, in sharp contrast to the prevalent policy of keeping it quiet. Kádár also announced that a monument was to be dedicated in Budapest in honor of Raoul Wallenberg, to be erected where his Swedish safe houses were located in 1944.

Eva and I had the opportunity to exchange a few words with Kádár. His relaxed, unpretentious manner stood in sharp contrast to the traditional pomposity of Hungarian politicians and the supercilious arrogance of the communist functionaries. We later had a long conversation with Kádár's physician, a medical school classmate of ours from Budapest in 1945 and 1946. I wanted very much to know what he thought of Kádár, who was willing to assume the role of the traitor, the heaviest burden you can carry before your people. How could he keep from becoming frightened, paranoid, and bitter? Why didn't he become one of those vacuous, isolated, misanthropic tyrants, the curse of so many oppressed nations? How could he maintain a positive attitude to such a degree that he became the most beloved figure in his country for a while, in the course of only a decade and a half?

Many stories and anecdotes circulated about Kádár in Hungary during his days of glory. According to one account, Kádár would easily have won 100 percent of the vote at one point in the 1970s, if the country had had a general election. Ninety percent of the people would have voted for him of their own free will, while the remaining 10 percent, would have been forced to do so by the discipline of the Communist Party to which they belonged. About 10 percent of the country's population were members of the party.

As our colleague noted, Kádár's most important personal characteristic was his ability to evaluate each situation by himself, listen to the advice of others, prepare himself thoroughly, and finally arrive at his own decisions.

While he always seemed, at least on the surface, to be following instructions from the Soviet Union, no one really knew what Kádár's true intentions were. They were only manifested in his actions.

After a few years under Kádár's leadership, people began to notice, first skeptically but later with increasing confidence, that Kádár's ambitions differed from those of a traditional communist leader. It was more important for him to satisfy the needs of the people than to abide by the ideological demands of the party. At the same time, he was fully aware that it was only possible to change the political system gradually. His silent maneuvering turned out to be realistic. It has led to the Hungarian version of "glasnost," long before "glasnost" appeared in Moscow. The Hungarian developments may have served as a test case for reform-minded politicians in the Soviet Union.

Listen to your own judgment, rather than follow instructions or ideology? Have the courage to make your own decisions—where had I heard that before? Sartre's autobiography came to mind.

"What is Kádár's family background?" I asked my colleague.

In Kádár's case, one can hardly talk about a real family background. He was the illegitimate son of a servant girl who worked very hard all her life. At the age of ten, János Kádár read everything he could get his hands on. He was completely self-taught. His career was filled with many years of perilous work in the illegal Communist Party, with prolonged periods of imprisonment and torture during both the fascist period and the Stalin epoch.

"One fatherless pays tribute to another tonight," I thought to myself. Even Raoul Wallenberg was fatherless. In truth, we don't know very much about him as a person. The little that we do know has become obscured by his fate and our wish to know what really happened to him, together with the legends that have inevitably grown up around him. I am flipping through a recently published collection of letters that the young Wallenberg wrote to his grandfather and guardian, Gustaf Wallenberg. I am amazed by the grandfather's great concern for Raoul's future, his meticulous planning for the boy in every detail. He took a very dim view of the "vanity and indolence" that he saw all around him in Stockholm, a place where people "had not learned to take life seriously." The grandfather's desire to watch over young Raoul's life may seem a little strange to today's readers, but it was quite common for the era and for his social milieu. "I am trying with the most affectionate care to shape your character," Gustaf Wallenberg wrote to his grandson. He often spoke about "self-discipline," which he regarded as one of the most important virtues.

Raoul's responses confirm this image of his grandfather. Raoul acquiesced to his grandfather's admonitions, even with respect to his social life. Even though the boy had chosen to become an architect rather than enter a career in business and economics as his grandfather had so carefully planned, Raoul time and again points out that he doesn't want to disappoint his grandfather, and his letters reveal only an obedient and well-behaved young man.

Raoul's letters also give strong evidence of his keen powers of observation, a high intelligence, and a refined sensitivity, portending nothing, however, of the astounding fate that was to befall him. It would be impossible to predict the incredible stamina to come. There are no signs of nonconformism, and he gives no reason to anticipate that his future behavior was destined to deviate in any way from established norms. These standards certainly included an immense respect for human values and democratic principles of justice, but Raoul's commitment to these values needn't have gone any further than mere verbal declarations among his own circle of friends, all of whom shared the same values. There was no reason why he had to take great personal risks to rescue victims of persecution, for it wouldn't have been difficult for him to formulate the usual rationalizations for avoiding such risks. He could easily have used a polished facade and glib arguments to hide a reluctance to become involved, out of fear or indifference. The understandable egoistic urge to put one's own career and safety before all else has always been the universally accepted norm, and Raoul's correspondence with his grandfather gives no indication that he would have behaved any differently. There is no reason to anticipate that Raoul would follow his own conscience at the risk of self-destruction, and it is all the more paradoxical and tragic that he not only did so, but also destroyed himself in the course of that process, although in a totally different way from what everybody had feared.

From a Swedish legalistic point of view, Wallenberg's intrepid rescue work was a clear transgression of his diplomatic powers. It would have been much easier for him to function within the limitations of what he was officially authorized to do. Other diplomats, also moved by humanitarian motives, might have limited themselves to issues of protective passports approved by the Swedish government for people with close relatives or at least with business connections in Sweden. Because of his desire go beyond these limits, Wallenberg succeeded in rescuing tens of thousands of people rather than only a few hundred. He obviously chose to act in accord with his own conscience, even though it clashed with diplomatic rules. He was not deluded by smokescreens or wishful thinking. He realized fully that he was dealing with a criminal, murderous regime. He knew the deportation trains were headed for death camps and not work camps, as was officially maintained. Many other diplomats and even statesmen chose to accept the lies of the Nazi regime, often against their better judgment.

Few are willing to sacrifice themselves for others. This is exactly what makes Raoul Wallenberg's actions unique. It is particularly depressing to compare Wallenberg's activity to the inactivity of the Swedish government after his disappearance. The contrast between these two attitudes is appalling—they are reciprocals of each other. In this case, the government was risking nothing, except possibly a slightly annoying diplomatic unpleasantness or an insignificant loss of prestige. Yet that became the determining factor. It was certain that Wallenberg was alive and in the Soviet Union after the war, despite vigorous denials by Soviet Foreign Minister Andrei Vyshinsky. The president of the Wallenberg Action Committee, Mrs. B. Bellander, visited the Swedish foreign minister, Östen Undén, in November 1948, and presented him with evidence that Wallenberg was still alive. When Undén asked if she believed Vyshinsky was lying, Mrs. Bellander answered that that was exactly what she believed.

"This is unheard of," Undén exclaimed, outraged, and thereafter he refused to have anything further to do with the matter. One must remember that the very same Vyshinsky was the public prosecutor in the Moscow purges and show trials that led to the false confessions and subsequent executions of so many leading revolutionaries during the 1930s. This was well known long before Mrs. Bellander's visit to Undén. That these confessions were criminal forgeries was always recognized by intellectuals in the Soviet Union. The official admission came when Gorbachev used the words "falsifications" and "fabrications" in his powerful speech to the party congress in October 1987.

Nevertheless, in 1947 the Swedish foreign minister preferred to believe the official Soviet version of the Wallenberg affair, delivered by the supreme forger of the show trials. He did so even though there was convincing evidence at the time that the Soviet answers were lies. When Undén declared that the Soviet government could not be presumed to be lying, he set the standard for later Swedish diplomatic behavior. This explains also why no one with a Wallenberg-like motivation appeared to attempt the rescue of the captured Raoul Wallenberg. One can possibly understand conformity, indifference, and caution among people in official or subordinate positions. It is exactly this everyday caution that conceals, in this case, the plain label of cowardice that makes Wallenberg's achievements so unique. But it is difficult to find any excuse for the paterfamilias behavior of the Swedish government, in this case. Even the otherwise super-correct and neutral Swiss were able to have their diplomats released from Russian captivity by playing the game the Russians obviously expected—that is, a bit of under-the-table horse trading. The result was an exchange of Swiss diplomats for Russian spies. Undén's haughty remark, aimed at the Swedish home audience, that the Swedish government doesn't barter with human beings seems to be nothing but a thin disguise for cowardice, conventional thinking, and fear of diverging from diplomatic etiquette. In negotiations with a criminal regime, one must forget one's good upbringing. A great burden of responsibility rests on the Swedish government for choosing to disregard the actions of the Stalin regime that were widely recognized as criminal by 1947.

What kind of people have I chosen to describe in this book? No, that's the wrong word—I haven't really chosen them—they have been stored in my memory for some reason. They have remained in one chamber or another, and I neither can nor want to let go of them. When I take a fresh look at them, I am suprised to find that several of them were fatherless, although I did not choose them on that basis. Was this sheer coincidence? One of them was Rudolf Vrba, who, together with his friend Wetzler, became the first to escape from Auschwitz and whose historical report of the death camp played such a major role in preventing the deportation of 200,000 Jews from Budapest. Two others are Edgar Allan Poe and Attila József, whose poetry has amazed, fascinated, and sustained me and millions of other readers for many years. Did the fact that they were fatherless contribute to their originality, as Sartre suggested? Is the escape of Vrba and Wetzler from Auschwitz the most dramatic and archetypically symbolic example of the ultimate existentialist choice?

In a recently published book,[3] D.K. Simonton provides extensive citations from the literature suggesting that the early loss of a father is disproportionately common among people noted for their exceptional scientific or literary achievements. Thirty percent of poets in one research study were fatherless.[4] According to another report,[5] one third of prominent people in many different professions had lost their father in early life. According to Simonton, there is a connection between fatherlessness, the development of independent thinking, an unconventional view of the world, and certain difficulties of social adaptability.

The question of how often the absence of an authoritative father figure can lead to criminal and antisocial behavior is also very interesting, but probably unanswerable. The link between fatherlessness and other frequently associated psychologically important factors such as broken families, economic deprivation, and the presence of a criminal environment might be too strong to allow meaningful analysis. An evaluation of the possible significance of individual factors in such complex cultural and environmental interactions is always difficult and may be quite impossible when both relevant parameters, fatherlessness and criminality, are relatively common. It is easier to discuss the possible role of fatherlessness in persons whose nonconformist behavior may be seen as an essential factor in relation to an exceptional achievement. My concluding example deals with a most unusual act in our times, deliberately chosen martyrdom.

The Austrian farmer Franz Jägerstätter was born 1907 in St. Radegund, a small village in Upper Bavaria, only twenty miles from Braunau-am-Inn, the birthplace of Hitler.[6] Linz, the capital of the province, was Hitler's favorite city, and he spent a great deal of his youth there. Adolf Eichmann also grew up in that city.

Jägerstätter's mother was unmarried. His biological father died during the First World War. His mother married the farmer Jägerstätter, who then adopted Franz, at the time only two years old. His illegitimate origin was common knowledge in the village, but there was no indication of any discrimination against him or his family. Franz grew up like other farm boys and was reputedly quite a wild young man, with a love for sports, dancing, card games, girls, and good fights. At one time he was a gang leader and was therefore involved in practically all the big fights in the neighborhood. Every once in a while he was arrested and forced to leave his village for a time, until the situation had calmed down a bit.

In 1936 he married a girl from a nearby village. The couple spent their honeymoon in Rome. As a result of the wedding or possibly shortly thereafter, Franz experienced a religious awakening. He was a Catholic by birth and attended Mass regularly, but after his return from Rome he became a fanatic believer. He observed all the religious doctrines and regulations, and, according to the villagers, stopped his drinking and card playing. He offered to help the priest as a volunteer sexton and served in that role with strict discipline. The villagers used to say that he stopped in at every church while out riding his motorcycle.

In 1938, Jägerstätter created a sensation by being the only one in his village to vote against the *Anschluss* (annexation) of Austria by Hitler's Germany. He openly declared that he considered the Nazis to be a gang of criminals. To the greeting "Heil Hitler!" he responded, "Pfui, Hitler!" It also became apparent that his aversion to socializing with the others at the local inn was based on motives other than religious ones—he simply wanted to avoid the endless political discussions.

Jägerstätter performed his obligatory military service from 1940 until 1941. His letters to his wife during this period reveal a growing dislike of the soldier's life. It was very difficult for him to put up with the drill, the irrational and arbitrary marching about, and the utter waste of time. His only solace was a hope that all this could impel him to a life of greater humility. He was also shocked by the cruelty of the soldiers toward their horses and other animals, and he asked his wife to send him sacks of special fodder. It was during his military service that he learned of the euthanasia program at a nearby mental hospital. Full of indignation and dismay, he wrote to his wife about the retarded little children who suddenly disappeared without a trace or who were announced to have died, overnight.

Although we don't know how much he knew about the Nazi program of genocide, it is possible that he was aware of the death camp at Mauthausen, because the trains ran near his village. Knowledge of these trains and of their human cargo must have been far more widespread than people were later willing to admit.

When he was drafted again in 1943, he refused to report for duty. By this time he already had three daughters, the oldest about six. He was sent to prison, first in Linz and later in Berlin. After he stubbornly refused to change his mind, he was sentenced to death by a military tribunal. On August 9, 1943, he was executed.

The American author and sociologist Gordon Zahn heard about Jägerstätter by pure chance during a vacation in Austria and became so interested that he undertook a systematic study of the story, finally publishing his findings in the book *In Solitary Witness*.[7] Jägerstätter's writings, published posthumously, include a number of short essays written shortly before his arrest, seventeen letters to his wife written while he was in prison, his farewell letters and a long explanation of his views that he wrote at the request of the prison chaplain. Zahn, himself a Catholic, also interviewed Jägerstätter's relatives, friends, acquaintances, and several Catholic priests who, in one way or another, were involved in his case. Zahn points out the pronounced contrast between Jägerstätter's religious conviction, which inspired him to follow his conscience and act without regard for the dangerous consequences, and the Catholic religious establishment, which was willing to adapt without raising any objections to the totalitarian state and its ruthless war.

In Zahn's view, the rebellious Jägerstätter personifies those who become martyrs through their nonconformist behavior. Zahn found that Jägerstätter's ideas and his determination could be traced to a time immediately after the war broke out. Although the family was hard-pressed economically, he handed out food and clothing to the poor. He urged other members in his congregation to boycott the Nazi relief organizations and give their support to acts of individual charity instead. He refused to accept either child support funds or any other agricultural or farmer's aid to which he was entitled from the state. On one occasion he reproached the village priest for praising the courage of a fallen soldier and calling his death heroic. For Jägerstätter this kind of glorification was irreconcilable with a truly religious outlook on life. He took a position distinctly opposed to that of his fellow Catholics and their church leaders, who accepted and often directly supported the war effort. In one of his essays he wrote, "How can one talk about defense of the Fatherland when you invade countries that owe you nothing, when you rob and murder there? What more can we Catholic Austrians lose if we no longer fight for the German state? Would we lose our religious freedom or our economic independence? . . . I cannot and never will accept the idea that we Catholics must make ourselves tools of the worst and most dangerous anti-Christian power that has ever existed."

His stand cannot be compared with that of those who resist the draft because of religious or pacifist attitudes. He would willingly have taken up arms if Austria had chosen to fight against Nazism. He writes with sympathy and with a certain envy about countries that dared to resist Nazi invasion. However, he never belonged to any organized resistance group. Available documents and witness statements are consistent in showing that he made his decision by himself. His starting premise was that the Austrians voluntarily capitulated to National Socialism in their acceptance of the Anschluss, and that the Catholic priesthood failed its collective conscience by not opposing Nazism firmly at that time. There were probably many individual priests who were opposed to the Anschluss and its implications, but who chose to remain quiet. The priest in St. Radegund, Pastor Joseph Karobath, argued that it would be pointless to vote against the Anschluss and that such an action would actually help the Nazis by identifying their potential opposition. Karobath also said that unanimous approval of the Anschluss would prove to the outside world that the election was forced upon them and that it did not truly reflect the will of the people. Jägerstätter did not accept this rationalization, especially since many other members of the clergy praised the Nazi party for its achievements, and in so doing increased its popularity. The acts of those priests strangled any chances for individuals to act according to their religious beliefs or to follow their own consciences, even if they had wanted to do so.

Without exception, the priests with whom Jägerstätter came into contact after he decided to refuse military service—including the highest local authority, the bishop of Linz—urged him to change his decision, to think first of his family and his own interests and let the leaders of the country decide what was politically right and wrong. A few priests expressed their admiration for Jägerstätter's unyielding will to follow his conscience all the way to the grave, but none of them gave him the support he needed most—the confirmation that he followed the right path in his actions. Zahn calls him a solitary witness, one who lacked any kind of external support at the moment of decision.

Among the comments of senior church officials, the reaction of the ordained bishop Fliesser of the diocese of Linz is the most interesting. This is the same bishop who repeatedly inhibited the full publication of Jägerstätter's story after the war. In his opinion, it would have been improper to discuss the case in a way that would "create confusion and disturb the consciences of the people." Zahn quotes the bishop's summary of his own evaluation:

I have known Jägerstätter personally, since he spent more than an hour with me before he answered the call for military duty. I explained for him the moral principles that limit the responsibility of the individual citizen in relation to the action of civil authorities. I reminded him that he had a much greater responsibility for his own life and for his family. I am aware of the "consistency" of his conclusions and respect their intention. At the time of our conversation, I could see that the man thirsted for martyrdom and for the expiation of sin, and I told him he was permitted to choose that path only if he knew he had been called to it through some special revelation originating from above and not from within himself. He agreed with this. For this reason, Jägerstätter represents a completely exceptional case. We may admire him, but should not try to emulate him. His case should be presented to the people only with this clear interpretation.

The most repulsive remarks in the bishop's letter are in the closing paragraph. He writes about "the young Catholic men, seminarians, priests, and head of families who fought and died in heroic fulfillment of duty and in the firm conviction that they were acting according to the will of God at their post . . . and are better models than the *Bibelforschers* (Bible scholars) and Adventists who . . . preferred to die in concentration camps rather than bear arms." It should be emphasized that this letter was written after the war and therefore could not have been the result of pressure from the Nazi regime or of fear of such pressure.

Zahn also interviewed Jägerstätter's defense counsel F.L. Feldmann, who had had many conversations with Jägerstätter in the Berlin prison before the execution. Jägerstätter was firm and unyielding. It was unthinkable for him to fight for the Nazi regime that was persecuting his Church and destroying its principles. When the lawyer pointed out that millions of other Catholics found it possible to do their duty for their nation even under such conditions, Jägerstätter replied simply, "They have not been granted grace." The counsel challenged him to cite a second instance in which a bishop, in either a pastoral letter or a sermon, had called upon Catholics not to support the war or to refuse military service. Jägerstätter admitted that he couldn't think of an example, but he added that this proved nothing other than the fact that they, too, had "not been granted grace." The attorney then quoted the Biblical injunction to "render therefore unto Caesar the things which are Caesar's," and asked by what authority Jägerstätter took a more "Catholic" position than the priests and bishops who had the responsibility of making theological judgments. Jägerstätter answered that he has made a moral judgment that could be made only by an individual conscience. When, in a final argument, the lawyer reminded Jägerstätter of his responsibilities toward his family, his client answered that his conscience must take precedence even over the most pressing personal considerations.

The trial took place on July 6, 1943. Feldmann describes a unique event that occurred shortly before the proceedings started. The room assigned for the trial was still in use, and Feldmann, his client, and two stern court officials of the military tribunal were forced to wait outside. The attorney pleaded desperately with the judges and described the sincere motives of his client, trying to enlist their informal help before the trial was to begin. They were accustomed to passing sentences over military deserters, and this case was unique for them. They listened to the lawyer and, departing from all tradition and practice, started an informal and initially very stern conversation with the accused. They asked if he was aware of the fate that was to befall him and his family if he continued to refuse service to his "Fatherland." Jägerstätter's answer was calm—yes, he was fully aware of the penalty, but he could not do otherwise. The argument progressed along all-too-familiar lines. The officers pointed out that individuals who had no access to information on secret military matters could not make competent judgments about the situation and the interests of the entire country. Jägerstätter's response was a calm and firm rejection of the arguments.

As the conversation progressed, Feldmann noted a distinct change in the tone of the military judges. At first they were stern and haughty, but their tone changed in the course of conversation. It was as if they had started, at first slowly and almost imperceptibly, to plead with the prisoner they were about to condemn. They appeared to look for a formula that could save them from the obligation of condemning him to death. Could he possibly accept some sort of noncombatant service in an office or a hospital, dressed in military uniform? No, it would be wrong, Jägerstätter said. He rejected all suggestions calmly but firmly.

Once they were all seated in the courtroom, the trial was short. Jägerstätter stood his ground, and after a short procedure, he was sentenced to death. Several priests saw him after the trial and before the execution. They all tried to dissuade him—he had only to sign a paper stating that had changed his mind, and his life would be spared. Up to the very last moment of his life, the written statement lay on the table in front of him, but he didn't sign it. His usual response was, "I cannot relinquish the responsibilities for my actions to Hitler." But who was Hitler if not the father figure for the misled German people? I recalled the German soldiers I met as I sat with my forged identification papers in the underground shelters in Budapest during the siege of the capital. They still managed to look quite neat in their uniforms, and did their utmost to convince one another that their Führer would keep his promises, that all was not yet lost, even at this late hour. The wonder weapon was sure to appear any day now—he had said so himself. German troops would no doubt liberate the encircled city very soon.

The determination to assume responsibility for his actions was a central feature of Jägerstätter's personality. In one of the essays left behind, he wrote:

It is often said that "it's alright for you to do this or that with an untroubled mind: the responsibility for what happens rests with someone else." And in this way responsibility is passed on from one man to another. No one wishes to accept responsibility for anything. Does this mean that one or two individuals will bear all the responsibility for the horrible crimes of our time on the say of the ultimate judgment?[4]

Of course it is very comforting to hear that others are responsible for our actions, but such assurances are unconvincing. Ultimately, you must be true to yourself.

On the night before Jägerstätter's execution, Chaplain Jochmann was on duty at the prison. The execution was scheduled for seven o'clock in the morning. Ordinarily the priest found the condemned prisoners in a state of panic and disorientation. But Jägerstätter was calm and prepared as Jochmann entered the cell. Not a word of complaint passed his lips. On the table in front of him lay the unsigned document. The priest made one last appeal and begged the prisoner to sign the paper that would free him. Jägerstätter pushed the document aside with a calm smile and said, "I cannot and will not take an oath to a government that is fighting an unjust war."

The priest offered several devotional booklets and asked if he wished to be read something from the New Testament. Jägerstätter declined, saying "I am in harmony with my own God. Books or listening to reading would only disturb that." The priest could never forget the expression of joy and self-confidence in the young farmer's eyes. He walked to the scaffold quietly, with the same expression.

It is late. Yes, father, I have nearly finished my essay on the fatherless. Are you wondering about the music we are listening to? It is Béla Bartók's "Cantata Profana," written three years after your death. Yes, you are quite right, it is the story of a father and his nine handsome sons who went into the woods to hunt. The sons followed the tracks of a large deer deep into the woods and became gradually transformed into deer. The father went to search for his sons—it was late, the table at home was already laid for supper, and the candles were lit. But instead of his sons, he found the nine deer. Just as he raised his rifle, his eldest son, the most handsome and most beloved, said, "Dear father, don't aim your gun at us. If you do, we will pierce you with our antlers, we will toss you from crag to crag, from rock to rock."

"Come with me, follow me home," said the father. "Your dear mother has supper ready, the candles are burning, the glasses are filled with wine."

"No, we will not come," answered the most handsome and most beloved of the sons. "Our feet can no longer tread and walk on floorboards, only on the leaves of the forest—our lips can no longer drink from crystal glasses, only from pure forest streams."

Is this the fate of a father? Is this the fate of the sons? I too am a father, but I have no father of my own. I no longer have the courage to put questions to my own son and daughters. But I would still like to meet you, father—I long to hear your voice. I would gladly sacrifice my power of initiative that people sometimes praise. I would relinquish my notorious self-assurance or arrogance—whatever it might be called. I would have given up my youth now long past, I would still give up my old age yet to come, to have met you just once, to listen to the sound of your voice. I would tell you all that has happened since you left us. Father, little brother, my son, my creator, you who will never allow me to know you, come, oppress me, crush me, mold me into whatever you want—into someone I never was, never will be, if only I could tell you that. . . . What would I really want to tell you? Perhaps only this: It is wonderful to live— thank you for making that possible for me. I probably would have killed you if you had lived, but I was never truly able to live while you were dead.

Part Five

7

Biological Individuality

Are you like me? Yes and no. From an everyday sociological perspective, we tend to take more notice of our differences. But from a biological point of view, we are very much alike. The functions of our cells rely on the same basic principles and utilize the same materials. Our hearts, our lungs, our kidneys perform their normal functions more or less identically. This is also reflected by our perception of the word "normal." We have come to expect that our basic functions will vary only within very narrow limits.

Can our cells function together if they are fused? Yes, without any difficulty. If you are a woman, my spermatazoa can fertilize your eggs and we can have a child together. If I fuse my tissues with yours, we can generate a functional hybrid cell. In spite of the fact that it has twice as many chromosomes as normal, it can survive and grow perfectly well in tissue culture. Our artificial creature can fill many plastic tissue culture dishes and provide as much material as cell researchers might need for analysis. Eventually it will lose some of its chromosomes; just as a balloonist throws bags of sand ballast overboard when he wishes to soar higher, the hybrid cell can afford to throw away unneeded loads. Each cell carries two copies of each specific chromosome, and the fused cell doesn't need four chromosomes of every kind. Chromosome loss occurs at random because the hybrid cell cannot distinguish between your chromosomes and mine.

The cells of our tissues are more tolerant of their fusion partner than our germ cells—spermatozoa or egg cells. I can hybridize any of my tissue cells with the cells of an ape, a mouse, or a rat, and the resulting mouse-human or rat-human hybrid cells are fully viable in tissue culture. However, the sandbags, the super-fluous chromosomes, are lost more rapidly and with unequal probability compared with the human-human hybrid cells. Human and mouse chromosomes do not replicate at exactly the same rate when they find themselves in the same hybrid cell. The human chromosomes are lost more often and more quickly. In a fusion between a mouse cell and a hamster cell, the mouse chromosomes are more quickly eliminated. This preferential elimination depends on the mechanics of chromosome move-ments during the process of cell division, which is slightly differ-ent in different species.

As long as human and mouse chromosomes are in the same hybrid cell, they can cooperate with each other without any difficulty. Defects, mutations, or partial losses that may have occurred in the chromosomes of one species can be readily compensated for by the partner, even if one is human and the other is mouse. This is called "genetic complementation." If one of my chromosomes contributes a function essential for the viability of the cell but whose counterpart on the mouse chromo-some has been damaged through a genetic accident, my chromo-some will be retained in the cell, even after my other chromo-somes are lost from the hybrid cell. This is due to the fact that my chromosome has become a "vital requirement" for the hybrid cell, because it provides a function that is essential for the cell's survival.

Can we exchange our tissues and whole organs, you and I? Yes and no. Without medical manipulation it is possible only if we are identical twins. In that case, there are no problems beyond the technical-surgical procedure itself. Your skin is my skin, your kidneys are my kidneys, your heart is my heart. You are I. From a genetic point of view, we are two copies of one individual.

If you are not my identical twin, my immune system will react against your tissues. My lymphocytes and macrophages, the two most important workhorses of the immune system, mount their attack within one or two weeks after they have come into contact with your transplanted cells. They need this "learning period" to draw the appropriate conclusions that you are not I. They are not comfortable with this arrangement and reject the guest cells.

They are not like a well-trained dog that can remain calm if that is the master's wish. They are implacably aggressive toward the foreign intruder. They destroy your cells whether you have given me just a small piece of your skin, some white blood cells, or an essential organ like a kidney or heart. Their eagerness to kill your cells may thus lead to their own and to my death—the rejection reaction runs its blindly suicidal course.

If it was a small piece of skin that has been rejected, we can easily try it a second time. Would the watchdogs get accustomed, would they have become more tolerant? No, on the contrary. The second rejection reaction occurs much more quickly, and no learning period in required. My "killer cells" are ready for you, they are hypersensitized against some substance you have that I lack. They prevent your skin from finding a foothold and attracting new blood vessels that could provide nourishment as it did the first time. Your skin cannot cover wounds on my skin even temporarily—it would be gone in two or three days. I can only accept tissue from you for a prolonged period of time if my immune system had been damaged earlier by treatment with drugs toxic to the immune system, with antiserum directed against my lymphocytes, or by radiation. In those cases, transplants can work quite well, providing that our tissues match each other relatively well. However, they can never match each other completely unless we are identical twins.

But what is meant by a "relatively good match"? Matching with respect to what? This is the key question of transplantation, but as we will see, its importance extends far beyond tissue transplantation. Before we examine this problem more closely, we must go back in history.

Long before the turn of the twentieth century, clinical experience had shown that tissue transplantation between humans results in a rejection reaction. A tissue transplanted between two individuals of the same species who are not identical twins is called a homograft, and the rejection is therefore called a *homograft reaction*. Many decades of this century had elapsed before it was realized that this is an immunological reaction, mediated by lymphocytes. It took several more decades before information became available on the nature of the lymphocyte's "target," or in other words, the molecules that set off the reaction. It was obviously a phenomenon of interactions between molecules that must vary among different individuals. But which gene or genes could be so widely polymorphic to make all individuals of a species different from each other? How could their products that were indigenous to the species elicit such strong immune reactions? Previously it was believed that strong immune reactions were reserved for foreign microorganisms, parasites, and proteins alien to the body.

Genetic analysis of tissue transplantation began in the wrong place for the wrong reason. It started in a cancer research laboratory focused on the study of hereditary factors in cancer development. Tissue transplantation was of no interest to the investigators there. But to perform the tumor studies, they grafted cancer cells from one animal to another to keep the cells alive, and they discovered the fundamentals of tissue transplantation as a by-product of this research. They found that the same principles govern the transplantability of normal cells and tumor cells. The rules derived from the relatively simple tumor transplantation experiments are still fully valid today.

The cancer geneticists wanted to determine if, and to what extent, hereditary factors contributed to the development of different kinds of tumors. It is very difficult to study this question in the human population because hereditary, cultural, and environmentally determined factors are intertwined. The methods of modern epidemiology can allow certain conclusions, but the clarification of hereditary influences is difficult, even today.

During the first three decades of the century, those working at the laboratory of Thomas Morgan at Columbia University in New York, more than any other group of scientists, made great progress in genetics. They chose the easily manipulated and rapidly reproducing fruit fly *Drosophila* as their main experimental object. Research with this apparently unpretentious and yet highly sophisticated creature has laid the foundation for much of modern genetics and molecular biology.

The geneticists realized very early that they had to work with highly inbred strains. After twenty or thirty successive brother-sister matings, they were able to derive "pure lines" consisting of genetically identical individuals that were essentially like a large collection of identical twins. Within such strains, all genes exist in only one form, and the father and mother transmit their identical sets of genes to every one of their offspring (not counting the Y-chromosome that exists only in the male). In standard scientific terminology, the strain is said to have become *homozygous*. To study the heredity of cancer, it appeared absolutely necessary to breed homozygous mammals. The smallest mammal is the obvious choice. The mouse, our evolutionarily closely related cousin, can produce three generations each year and it is susceptible to many forms of cancer that are more or less similar to human tumors.

Thirty brother-sister matings over a period of ten years were required before the first strains were ready at the beginning of the 1930s. But the results were well worth the trouble. From the very beginning, the inbreeding program included selection for or against susceptibility to cancer. The important question was whether the inbred offspring from a female who had developed breast cancer would have an increased incidence of the same tumor if the offspring of mothers who later developed breast cancer were selected in each generation for breeding. Conversely, would the strain become cancer-free if mice that had reached old age and remained free of cancer were selected as the parents of later generations? Both questions were answered in the affirmative. Subsequent studies have shown that the propensity of the mice to develop breast cancer was influenced by hereditary and viral and hormonal factors. This is a separate issue, and I wish here to concentrate on the transplantation experiments.

Before inbred animals became available, it was thought that only a small fraction of all mouse tumors could be transplanted from one animal to another. Most transplants did not grow. Therefore, a distinction was made between transplantable and nontransplantable tumors. This interpretation, however, was spurious, because when the transplantation experiments were repeated with tumors that had appeared in the inbred strains, *all* tumors could be transplanted to mice from the *same* strain. There the cells continued to grow until they killed the recipient animals. In mice of a different strain, they also began to grow, but after several days or weeks the tumors decreased in size and eventually disappeared. The sequence of events corresponded to what had been seen after transplantation of normal tissues, with the exception that the transplanted cancer cells were able to grow temporarily in the new host animal. Microscopically, the same reaction was seen in both cases; the graft of transplanted cells was invaded by the host's lymphocytes, directly destroying the foreign cells and also damaging the vascular system of the graft.

These experiments led to the *first law of transplantation*, which states that malignant as well as normal tissues are freely transplantable between genetically identical individuals within an inbred strain and between identical twins, but are rejected by genetically foreign recipients.

The so-called transplantable tumors mentioned earlier that were not impeded by this genetic transplantation barrier and could grow even in foreign strains were in reality genetic variants that might be compared to antibiotic-resistant bacteria. Either they were resistant to the rejection reactions and/or they grew so rapidly that the reactions of the host animal were not able to keep up. Most of these "nonspecifically transplantable tumors" have been established in the laboratory by a series of selective passages. In the beginning, the foreign recipients were quite resistant, but the removal and further transplantation of the temporarily growing tumors eventually led to the establishment of variants that grew in virtually all foreign recipients of the same species. The ability of the tumor cells to surmount the transplantation barriers could increase from several percent to 100 percent after prolonged passage of the cells.

But tumor cell variants of this kind could also occasionally appear without any laboratory selection. One spontaneous variant of this type acquired a natural mode of transmission. The "venereal sarcoma" of dogs is the only cancerous disease that can be transferred sexually by cell transplantation. One single strain of cells with distinctive chromosonal and other characteristics is transmitted by sexual intercourse in dogs in Europe, Japan, and the United States. The possibility that such an unusual cell strain will appear is very low, and the likelihood that it could become sexually transmitted is almost completely nil. Nevertheless, this doubly improbable event has actually occurred in a mammalian species. The tumor is not especially malignant, because its cells are more foreign to the host than the host's own cells. Immunization with killed tumor cells can protect the dogs. In contrast, immunization of an individual against tumor cells that have originated in itself or in animals that have the same genetic constitution, like identical twins or other members of the same inbred strain, can provide only weak or no immunity.

Following the discovery of the first law of transplantation, genetic methods have been used to obtain information about the genes that regulate the rejection reaction. When two inbred strains, A and B, were crossed and the offspring grafted with tumor cells from one parental strain, the tumors of both the A and B strains grew freely in mice of the first hybrid generation (F_1). It was concluded that the ability of the tumor to grow after transplantation was determined by dominant genes, designated as "histocompatibility" (tissue compatibility) genes or H-genes. Because both the parent strains were highly inbred, all their genes, including the H-genes, were present in two identical copies in each strain. In other words, the mice were homozygous for those genes. Their F_1 hybrids were heterozygous, but all F_1 hybrids from a given cross were genetically identical and showed none of the variations normally found among ordinary siblings in noninbred strains. Every gene of each F_1 hybrid was present in every individual of one or the other parental strain. The only difference is that the hybrids contain only single copies of each of the genes from the A and B strains, whereas the parents contain two copies of each gene. Because every F_1 hybrid offspring contained all the genes from every potential tumor donor of both parental strains, they could not reject the tumors or normal tissues from either the A or B strain. Such a rejection reaction would be like a reaction against oneself.

The *second law of transplantation* states that F_1 hybrid offspring of two inbred strains are susceptible to the transplantation of tissues from both parents.

The expression "tissue compatibility" was coined before it was clear that the rejection was caused by the immune response of the host. If that had been known, they could just as well have been called "tissue incompatibility genes." The rejection reaction is directed against the foreign H-gene products in the grafted tissue. H-genes vary in the population just like blood group genes, but they occur in considerably more diverse forms.

How many different H-genes exist? That question was studied by two further types of genetic crosses, designated as F_2 and backcross hybrids, respectively. An F_2 hybrid is derived from the cross between two F_1 hybrids of the same type. A dominant characteristic that is determined by a single gene, such as hair color, eye color, blood group or, as in the present case, the ability to reject grafts, occurs in 75 percent of the F_2 offspring.

If F_1 hybrids between strains A and B, where A is susceptible and B is resistant to the grafting of tumors from A, are backcrossed to the resistant B parent, 50 percent of the offspring will accept strain A tumors. This expectation was confirmed experimentally. Tumors that "require" the presence of one dominant H-gene from the A strain of origin grew in 75 percent of the A x B F_2 hybrids and in 50 percent of the A x B F_1 backcrosses to B.

Let us now suppose that a tumor can grow progressively only if two different genes, H-1 and H-2, are identical with the host. The probability that the F_2 offspring contain both these genes in the same form as the A strain is three fourths of three fourths, or 56 percent. Half of half, or 25 percent, of the backcross hybrids contain both genes in the A form. When dealing with three genes, the incidence becomes $(3/4)^3$ or 43 percent in the F_2 hybrids, or $(1/2)^3$ or 12.5 percent in the backcrosses.

By determining the frequency of animals susceptible to the grafting of the same tumor in the F_2 hybrids compared with the backcrosses, it is possible to determine the number of genes that the tumor and the host must share to prevent a rejection reaction. After such comparisons were made on a larger material, it turned out that the "matching requirements" of different tumors were different. Some could grow if one critical gene was present in the recipient, whereas others required a match of two, three, or even more genes.

In experiments with normal tissues, the compatibility requirements were even greater. Fifteen or more genes had to be matched for full acceptance. It was becoming obvious that it was more important to match some genes than others. This has led to the concept of strong and weak H-gene barriers. Tumors could transgress weak barriers quite easily, particularly if they grew to a large size before an efficient reaction started. Normal tissues were often rejected by weak barriers as well, however, because they did not grow progressively but had to remain in their proper place and carry out their function.

After a large number of tumors had been tested, it became obvious that there was only *one* strong gene that had to be matched in most cases. Only the "transplantable" tumor variants described above were able to grow in the absence of such matching. The same gene also provided the fastest and most powerful barrier against transplantation of normal tissues. Its importance is reflected in its name, *major histocompatibility complex,* or MHC. Today's clinical transplantation practices require the best possible MHC matching. The viral H-genes are ignored, because their function can be weakened by drugs that suppress the immune system.

Transplant donors and recipients can be matched for MHC to various degrees. This is determined by the availability of suitable donors and also by the relative vulnerability of the tissues involved. A bone-marrow transplant must be matched as exactly as possible because the recipient patient is doubly vulnerable. The bone marrow contains the lymphocytes (one type of white blood cells) that trigger or mediate immune responses. Two opposed immunological reactions may occur between an incompletely matched bone marrow and its host. One is the host's reaction against the transplant, and the other the transplant's reaction against the host. The latter is particularly dangerous and can lead to the potentially lethal "graft versus host disease." A complete MHC match is therefore more important for bone-marrow transplants than for kidney or other organ transplants where only the host reacts against the graft. A sibling who has inherited the same two MHC genes from father and mother as the recipient is the preferred donor for a bone-marrow transplant. This situation is found with a probability of 25 percent (one in four siblings). There are no ethical problems with this choice, because the bone-marrow donor does not suffer any permanent tissue loss.

Kidney transplantation poses a somewhat greater ethical dilemma. A donor can manage quite well with only one kidney, but obviously loses a potentially important reserve organ. In these cases, the principles of medical ethics demand that siblings not be asked to serve as donors and not even be typed as potential donors. The reason for this is easy to see. The chance that two siblings would be completely MHC identical are 25 percent, as already mentioned, because the MHC genes of the parents can be recombined in four different ways. If we designate the two MHC-carrying chromosomes of the father as AB, and those of the mother as CD, then their children can be AC, AD, BC, or BD. The probability that any two siblings would both become AC is one in four, or 25 percent. Identification of the most appropriate, fully MHC-matched sibling would result in such a great burden on the potential donor that "donation" of the organ could not be regarded as truly voluntary. A biologically less satisfactory solution has been found that is fully acceptable from an ethical point of view. In most developed countries, healthy kidneys from MHC-compatible accident victims are being used for transplantation. Matching is performed only for the most easily identifiable MHC "flags," that is, gene products in the huge MHC complex. The entire complex is too large to be identical in two separate and unrelated individuals. Two siblings with the same MHC-carrying chromosomes from both father and mother are identical over the entire complex. The priority of ethical over medical considerations in this case provides an interesting example of medical ethics at work.

The road toward today's efficient transplantation methods has been a long one. By the 1940s, one of the "founding fathers" of the field, George Snell, had already formulated the laws of transplantation described above. Several years later, the Englishman Peter Gorer discovered that rejection of tissues between genetically different mouse strains is accompanied by the production of antibodies that can destroy the white blood cells of the donor strain in the test tube. Fortunately, the antibodies were not directed against all or even most of the H-gene products mentioned above, but only against the strong rejection-mediating MHC proteins. It was therefore possible to develop a relatively simple MHC typing method that opened the way for the clinical application of this originally purely experimental research with mice.

Human tissue typing began toward the end of the 1950s, when the Frenchman Jean Dausset transplanted small pieces of human skin to experimental subjects. Following the rejection of the foreign skin, the recipients were found to develop antibodies that could kill the donor's lymphocytes in the test tube. Similar antibodies could be demonstrated in people who had received many blood transfusions and in women who had had many children. Pregnant women are immunized by the fetal cells that reach the mother's blood circulation early in pregnancy. The maternal antibodies are directed against the MHC proteins derived from the father. The fetus itself—nature's own transplant—is protected from the mother's antibodies and killer lymphocytes in different ways. Just as in the case of many other essential processes such as blood coagulation or the regulation of the body's thermostat, the mammalian fetus is protected by a variety of different mechanisms. They shelter it from the rejection reaction that would effectively remove other foreign tissues. Many groups of scientists have studied these mechanisms. Each of them had its own favorite theory about "the" mechanism responsible for fetal protection. It turned out, however, that practically all mechanisms you could think about were actually at work in one form or another. The fetus is protected against penetration by the mother's killer lymphocytes by mechanical and biochemical barriers. The fetus minimizes its own release of MHC that would immunize the mother by the interposition of an MHC-free layer of cells on the side of the placental surface facing the maternal cells. Just in case this would not be sufficient, maternal rejection reactions against foreign transplants are generally impaired during pregnancy. These are only some examples of the many potentially relevant mechanisms that have been demonstrated. The continuation of a normal undisturbed pregnancy and the eventual birth of immunologically undamaged offspring are of such central evolutionary significance that all mechanisms that might possibly contribute to the protection of the fetus have obviously been fixed by natural selection.

At this point one may ask why the rejection reaction has been retained at all during evolution. Wouldn't it have been simpler to eliminate it entirely rather than to accumulate so many complicated protection mechanisms for the fetus? Because transplantation of foreign cells does not pose any serious dangers, why is the rejection reaction so strong against cells that differ only with respect to their MHC markers? Why is it that the reaction against other genetically variable proteins, including the weak H-gene products, is so comparatively unimportant? There is only one logical answer to this question: the "recognition" of MHC proteins is at least as important as the mechanisms protecting the fetus! Even without the experimental evidence that I will describe shortly, it is easy to understand that the MHC-mediated rejection reaction must have a fundamental biological significance, because it is equally well developed in fish, birds, reptiles, and amphibians as it is in mammals. It is therefore evolutionarily older than viviparity, the birth of living young in mammals. Similar rejection mechanisms are found among invertebrates, although they are not directly comparable to the MHC system.

Before we delve more deeply into the state of the art, I want to go back to the end of the 1950s. Jean Dausset and the Dutchman Jan van Rood showed that humans can produce cell-killing antibodies against white blood cells from foreign donors just as well as mice. But did the antibody reactions in the humans and mice really correspond to each other? A great deal was already known about the MHC system of mice and about its genetics, but nothing was known about the possible existence of MHC genes in humans. The first important piece of information came from the skin transplantation experiments of Dausset, mentioned earlier. His attempts to gather volunteers for the skin-grafting experiment became a great success from the scientific perspective and also from a broader psychological and sociological point of view. Dausset's personality and his remarkable ability to explain his experiments contributed to this great success. He regularly assembled the volunteers to explain the goals of the work and to report the latest results. He even organized Christmas parties for their families. He was able to convey his scientific excitement to them. It was clear to all volunteers that their contribution, which caused them only slight discomfort, helped science to make important advances in a previously uncharted territory and offered the hope of important practical applications in the future. And so it was to be.

With the help of the cell-killing antibodies from the transplanted volunteers, Dausset was able to work out a preliminary classification of the corresponding antigens in the human population. Parallel studies by van Rood in Holland on women who had had multiple births was providing similar information. The family studies of these women showed that the protein or proteins eliciting the antibody responses were inherited through a single gene, localized on a precisely defined chromosome of the chld's or the children's father. That indicated that humans could also have an MHC system similar to that found in the mouse. But the workers were very cautious at the outset. The human system was called HLA, or "human leucocyte antigen," because it was still not known if the antigen—the target for the antibody on the cell membrane—existed only on the white blood cells that were destroyed by the antibodies, or if they were also present on all other cells, like the mouse MHC antigens. Kidney transplantation, which had been started at many surgical centers by this time, provided the answer. Tissue typing, based on the killing of white blood cells of the donors and the recipients by the HLA antibodies, turned out to be relevant for predicting the fate of the transplants. Differences in the HLA markers produced strong rejection reactions, while matched HLA markers were associated with better survival of the transplanted tissue.

In more recent years, we have come to realize that the human system is completely analogous to that of the mouse. Today's advanced molecular methods have proved that the two systems "talk" almost the same DNA language. It is like reading the same text in Swedish and Norwegian. One can say that the MHC genes are highly conserved. The evolutionary step from mouse to humans has produced only minor differences among them.

Does the Rejection Reaction against Foreign Transplants Reflect a Normal Immunological Function?

Genes that have been highly conserved by evolution are usually referrred to as "housekeeping" genes. They play a fundamental role in the life of all cells. What could be the function of the MHC system? It had been discovered through the rejection of foreign grafts, which is an experiemental artifact in itself. It gives no direct information about the normal physiological function of the system.

One of the most characteristic features of the system is its polymorphism, or diversity. It exists in alternative forms in different people. What role can the MHC genes and their products play in a normal individual who is not being confronted with a tissue graft? What advantage does the polymorphism provide to the species?

Our knowledge of the system has evolved slowly and gradually, and is still incomplete, but by 1980 it was sufficiently well developed to earn the Nobel Prize for the discoverers of the mouse and human systems, George Snell and Jean Dausset. A third immunologist, Baruj Benacerraf, was included for his studies on the function of the system.

The products of the MHC complex had previously been identified as well-defined protein molecules located within the membranes of cells. This was achieved with the help of the antibodies described above. The first indication that these molecules can play an important role in immunological reactions in a normal organism came from the study of so-called killer cells that destroy normal and malignant cells in culture. The killer cells were first identified by virtue of their role in the rejection of foreign transplants, as already mentioned. Later studies have generated results of much greater importance, however. Their impact extended far beyond transplantation research. It became more and more apparent that the MHC system affects all cell-mediated immune responses in the intact organism.

In the original experiments aimed at transplantation problems, lymphocytes were mixed from two strains of mice differing at their MHC gene locus. This has led to a mini-rejection reaction in the test tube. A certain type of lymphocyte, the so-called T-cell, could react against foreign lymphocytes whose own reactivity had been inhibited by previous irradiation or drug treatment, to avoid confusion. The reactive T-cells increased in size and then began to divide and replicate. Some of the newly produced cells were very effective at killing the foreign cells. They were dubbed CTL (cytotoxic T-lymphocytes) or, in other words, killer cells. These cells literally punched holes in the membranes of the target cells, a dramatic "kiss of death" that could be seen and photographed in the microscope. The killer cell resembles a hand mirror. It touches the target cell with the "mirror handle." Soon thereafter, the movements and other vital functions of the prey come to a quick halt. The killer cell survives and moves on to continue its war against additional target cells.

When the CTL cells were mixed with target cells from foreign strains that had the same MHC gene as the CTL cells themselves, but differred with respect to other H-genes, the "kiss of death" did not take place. But if the donor mice of the CTLs had been pre-immunized against these weaker H-gene products, the killer cells could recognize and kill MHC-identical target cells that carried the same weaker H-genes against which the donor had been immunized. The question arose whether ordinary antigens from the environment, including substances that produce allergies, could also function as targets for immunized killer cells. The antigens were coupled chemically to target cells that were genetically identical with the potential killer cells. These CTL cells were taken from donors who had been immunized against the antigen. They were able to recognize their chemically modified target cells and apply their kiss of death to them, but not to corresponding unmodified target cells. This was interesting in itself, but a great surprise came from one of the control experiments. There was no killing when the chemical substance against which the CTLs had been immunized was coupled to a target cell whose MHC differed from the MHC of the CTL cells! Other T-cells would probably have reacted gradually against the foreign MHC components on these target cells, but the pre-immunized CTL cells did not. The process of pre-immunization had selectively enriched those T-cells that were able to react against the immunizing chemical antigen at the cost of other T-cells.

These experiments have led to the discovery of a new phenomenon. Specific immunological reaction could only take place if the killer cell and the target cell were completely or, as it was later shown, partly identical with respect to the MHC genes. Complete matching was not necessary. The same rule also applied to CTL cells immunized against the weaker H-gene products, as discussed earlier. Such CTLs could kill target cells that carried the weak H-antigens against which they had been immunized, but only if the killer cells shared MHC components with their target cells. This restriction of the reaction to MHC-matched target cells was called "MHC restriction." The concept of restriction implies that immunized lymphocytes recognize the antigen against which they have been immunized only if it is attached to or presented together with the lymphocyte's own MHC molecules (self-MHC). The question of how T-cells recognize foreign MHC became less interesting. It was a side phenomenon—a product of a laboratory experiment. The important question was how killer lymphocytes and other cells of the immune system made use of their own MHC to recognize the targets against which they had been immunized. The reaction against foreign MHC genes has come to be regarded as a secondary consequence.

The importance of MHC restriction became especially apparent in connection with immunological reactions against virus-infected cells. T-cells play a decisive role in the immune defense against viral infection. It is no coincidence that immunological disorders that affect the T-cells often lead to the eruption of latent virus infections. The reaction of T-cells against virus-infected cells is set off by the foreign viral proteins produced by the infected cells. But in contrast to what was previously thought, the T-cells do not "see" the viral proteins directly. They see only certain breakdown products that have been "chewed" off from these proteins in the infected cells, where they have become attached to newly produced MHC molecules and then transported to the membrane of the target cell. The T-cell itself must carry the same MHC molecules. Accordingly, the immunized T-cells react against a target structure that can be written "self + X," where "self" indicates the cell's own MHC molecules and X is a chemical substance, or a virally or genetically determined protein, or more precisely, its breakdown product.

T-cells can even protect against the growth of certain tumors. Virus-induced tumor cells are the most suitable targets, since they produce foreign viral proteins. Tumors that appear without any viral involvement often fail to induce any rejection reaction. This explains why virus-induced tumors usually appear in people with defects in their immune system. Normally, such "would-be tumor cells" are eliminated by the host response before they have had time to grow to a visible size. Infections that preferentially strike people with immune defects are called "opportunistic" infections, and similarly caused tumors are called "opportunistic" tumors. Both kinds of diseases take advantage of the immune failure by plundering their hosts with impunity.

The Significance of the MHC System for the Interaction between Cells of the Immune System

The new area of research opened through the discovery of MHC restriction has placed the MHC genes and their products among the most important target and regulatory structures for a large variety of immune responses. In addition to the cell-killing reaction between lymphocytes and their target cells, the MHC system also plays an important role in the interactions among other cells of the immune system.

Interactions between different cells of the immune system play a similar role in immunology as signal transmission between the cells of the nervous system. This is reflected by the frequently used expressions "immunological network" or "immunological orchestra." Unlike the nervous system, cells of the immune system do not use electrical or chemical signals. At least ten proteins have now been identified that instruct the cells of the immune system when to reproduce, when to make special materials such as killer substances or other products such as antibodies or new signal substances, when to lie low, and when to die. There is probably a whole forest of such signal substances still to be identified.

The three main categories of cells in the immune system are macrophages ("eaters of large particles"), T-lymphocytes, which mature in the thymus gland (hence the designation T-cell) and the B-lymphocytes that are produced in the bone marrow. The interaction between the macrophages and the T-cells provides the start signal for most immunological reactions. The macrophage "presents" the foreign protein that it has "eaten" and "digested" to the T-cell. Amazingly enough, this presentation is also mediated by the MHC system. But the MHC products that participate in this interaction are not the same as those in the cell-killing reaction. The killer cells interact with the so-called class I antigens, while the macrophages make use of another MHC component, the so-called class II antigens. The two classes of proteins are produced from the same large gene cluster or complex and are chemically similar. Class II molecules have their own restriction: macrophages and T-cells must match for at least part of their class II molecules to make the T cell "interested" in the breakdown product of the foreign protein presented to it by the macrophage.

When a macrophage presents the broken-down protein to the MHC class II-matched T-cells, only a small minority of the T-cells reacts. The match of MHC antigens is thus necessary but not sufficient to induce a reaction. All T-cells in a given individual have the same MHC components, but they also carry another membrane component, the T-cell receptor (TCR), which differs among different T-cells, and even *within* a given individual. TCR diversity is similar to the diversity of antibodies produced by the B-lymphocytes. The TCR molecules carried on the T-lymphocytes are related to the antibodies and belong to the same gene superfamily, but they are controlled by different genes. The two systems are adapted to "recognize" as many different antigens as possible.

Only a minority of T-cells stimulated by a given antigen carry a TCR molecule that fits the antigen, much like a lock for a certain key. The fragment of antigen presented by the macrophage really functions like an ignition key, but only under the double condition that it fits the TCR lock and that it is presented by an appropriate class II antigen on the macrophage that matches the T-cell's class II antigen. If both conditions are met, the process of cell division is induced, which leads to a rapid enrichment of the T-cells that can react against the antigen.

GOD (Generation of Diversity) in the Immune System

T-cell receptors and antibodies diversify in a given individual through essentially the same mechanism. GOD, the "generation of diversity" in the immune system remained enigmatic for many years and was the favorite area for speculations. More recently, GOD has lost its mystery and had been reduced to DNA chemistry. Before looking more closely into this question, let us review quickly the three kinds of diversity that we must consider: variations in the configuration of the MHC proteins, the T-cell receptors, and immunoglobulins (antibodies).

Within an individual, MHC products exist in a limited number of different forms—about a dozen or so. Their DNA codes are carried by the chromosomes inherited from the parents, one from the father and one from the mother. The entire MHC text is written in exactly the same form in all cells of the body, although only certain parts are used to produce proteins in all cells. Other regions are only active in some tissues. MHC is enormously variable between individuals, but not within an individual. In contrast, the immunoglobulins and the T-cell receptors occur in an enormous number of different forms within each individual. Each person can therefore react to hundreds of thousands, or possibly even to millions, of different substances. The T-lymphocytes recognize these substances, or rather their digested breakdown products, by means of their T-cell receptors (TCR), as already mentioned.

B-lymphocytes carry their antibody product on their outer membrane. The cells are activated to divide when their antibody product "catches" the corresponding antigen. Antigen breakdown products are usually presented to the B-cells by T-cells. This interplay is also subject to the rules of class II restriction. The selective enrichment of B-cells that produce antibody against a triggering of antigen leads to a rise of the corresponding antibody level in the serum. These unbelievably sophisticated tools permit us to handle the innumerable foreign substances we are steadily confronted with from the microbiological world, the flora and fauna, and the synthetic products of human activities. We can make antibodies against many chemicals that our species has never encountered before during our evolution—because they did not exist before the development of modern industries. This "foresight" of the immune system is based on the enormous diversification of the T-cell receptor and immunoglobulin genes that occurs in all individuals from early fetal life.

The discovery that the diversity of the immunoglobulin genes is caused by continuous rearrangement of their DNA in the B-lymphocyte population earned the Nobel Prize for Susumu Tonegawa in 1987. Other workers showed later that the TCR genes also undergo similar rearrangements in the T-lymphocytes. These results came as a surprise, as they violated the old dogma that all cells in the body contain exactly the same DNA. It was thought that the maternally and the paternally derived DNA replicated in exactly the same form as they were present immediately after their first fusion in the fertilized egg cell. This rule is still valid for all cells outside the immune system. The great variety of tissue types results from a functional diversification of cells rather than from genetic, DNA-based variations. Specialized cells of the body "open different windows" on the same DNA building; liver cells, muscle cells, kidney cells all produce their specialized products by utilizing different parts of the same genetic material.

Immunoglobulin (Ig) and T-cell receptor genes become diversified, however, through a precisely controlled Monte Carlo game at the level of the DNA itself. They contain "hypervariable" regions that are rearranged in thousands of different combinations during the maturation of the lymphocytes. The gigantic "locksmith" constantly generates an enormous number of different "locks," so that every incoming "key" (each antigen) has a good chance of finding its own best fitting "lock."

The Immunological Orchestra

We may now recapitulate how the different pieces of the immunological jigsaw puzzle fit together. An antigen that enters an organism is first modified by the macrophages that serve as "ruminants" to offer well-chewed antigens to the T-cells. The rare T-cells that contain the best-fitting three-dimensional TCR (the lock) for that antigen respond to the invitation by accepting some of its pieces. Their own class II MHC molecules play an essential but incompletely understood role in this process. The encounter between the antigen and the corresponding TCR stimulates the T-cell to divide. The responding T-cell becomes selectively enriched. It expands preferentially at the expense of its unselected siblings. One type of T-cell, the *CD4* or *helper cell*, transfers the antigen fragment to the small minority of B-cells that are competent, due to their own immunoglobulin gene rearrangements, to produce an antibody that binds to that antigen. This binding activates the B-cells and stimulates them to divide and to produce antibodies. CD4 cells are the most important targets for the HIV virus (see the following chapter on AIDS). Another type of T-cell is transformed into the *killer* or *CD8* cells already described above, the cells that can destroy virus-infected cells or tumor cells that carry an antigen against which the lymphocyte has been immunized. Both the helper- and killer-cell functions are dependent on complete or partial MHC identity between the cells that "pass the ball," the antigen fragment, to each other (the T- and B-cells with respect to the MHC class II antigens, which participate in the helper function, and to T-cells and antigen-bearing target cells with regard to MHC class I antigens, which play an essential role in the killer function).

Diversity of the MHC System Protects the Species against Major Epidemics

The exact relationship of the antigen fragment to the MHC molecules has been enigmatic for a long time. Recent evidence from X-ray crystallography has now provided an answer. It is now one of the clearest and most beautiful facts in immunology. As so often in evolution, the precise adaptation of the system to its purpose is flabbergasting.

The MHC molecules carry on their outer surfaces a small ledge at the bottom of the groove, not far from the outer surface. The digested fragment is introduced into the groove and becomes attached to the ledge. The fragment is a peptide, a small breakdown product of the full protein that consists of eight or nine protein building blocks, or amino acids. The many different forms of MHC, carried by different individuals, differ in their ability to bind a certain peptide. The enormous polymorphism of the MHC system, its variation between different individuals in mammalian species, suggests that this variability may provide some advantage to the species. This may relate to this difference in binding. The total MHC repertoire of each person has a characteristic, individual pattern. Consequently, each individual will bind a somewhat different spectrum of peptides to their MHC molecules. This means that people differ with regard to their ability to react against the same antigen. Therefore, the variability of the MHC system offers an immunological flexibility to the species that can be of great value at the time of major epidemics. The importance of this flexibility becomes even more apparent if you consider the enormous capacity of bacteria, viruses, and parasites to change. They can readily generate new mutants, some of which may be better suited to escape the host immune response than the original form. The great influenza epidemics are examples of this kind of phenomenon. The many alternative forms of the MHC molecules increase the survival chances of a species, because they broaden its ability to react to epidemics compared with the limited repertoire of any individual. In other words, the variability of the MHC system enhances the preparedness of the species against hazards from the unknown.

What happens when a species is stricken with a great new epidemic? Does an individual with a certain MHC type fare better than others? One of the pioneers of the MHC system, Jan van Rood, has tried to approach this question by searching for significant gaps in the MHC repertoire of a well-defined immigrant group more than a century after it was devastated by two epidemics. He examined the distribution of MHC types among the living descendents of Dutch colonists who emigrated to Surinam in 1845 compared to the descendents of the same village that stayed in their homeland.[1]

The original emigrant group consisted of 367 people in 50 unrelated families. They left for South America to establish a farming colony. Two weeks after their arrival, they were stricken with a typhoid outbreak. Every person became ill, and 49 percent died. Six years later, 20 percent of the survivors died from yellow fever. Between and after these epidemics, the mortality rate was quite low. The survivors and their offspring remained in Surinam and married more or less only among themselves. Efficient family registration made it possible to trace the survivors' offspring accurately and to compare the presence of twenty-six different MHC variants in them with the offspring of their counterparts in Holland, who were spared the epidemics. Clear differences were found. Certain MHC components occurred in a higher frequency, others in a lower frequency among the offspring of the emigrants, indicating that the immunologically less reactive MHC types may have been eliminated, while more resistent MHC types may have survived in a selective fashion.

The investigators concluded that resistance against disease-producing microorganisms varied with the MHC type, in agreement with knowledge derived from studies on experimental animals. In another study, the same group found a connection between the production of antibodies against certain parasites such as malaria and the MHC type.[2]

One of the discoverers of MHC restriction, the Swiss scientist Rolf Zinkernagel, has found that most of the currently prevalent MHC types in any given mammalian species are associated with a high reactivity against the naturally occurring viruses of that species. Only a few variants demonstrated a low reactivity. They were often classified as immunologically "defective," ignoring the fact that the lack of reactivity applied only to certain very specific viral antigens. Quite a different result was obtained with disease-producing viruses that a species does not normally encounter in its natural habitat. Most of the MHC types were associated with a low reactivity, while only a few were highly reactive. In an epidemic, the highly reactive types would have a selective survival advantage.

Zinkernagel ascribes the inability of individuals with certain MHC types to respond to specific antigens as the "black hole of the immune repertoire." One type of black hole is unavoidable. It is the price we must pay for the vitally important phenomenon of "immunological tolerance"—the inability to reject our own tissues, the acceptance of "self." During fetal life, the immunological system "learns" to distinguish between "self" and "not self." T-cells that have developed an ability to react against the organism's own antigens by the TCR diversification process are continuously eliminated through a selection process that takes place in the thymus gland, one of the major "graveyards" of the immune system. This "education" of the T-cells takes place during embryonic life. If foreign cells are introduced into a fetus during this period, the fetus becomes "immunologically tolerant" to them. The system is fooled into regarding them and all their progeny cells as "self."

Due to this tolerance to "self" antigens, the organism may run into difficulties in recognizing foreign antigens that are quite similar to "self." The black holes are more gray than black, however. In most cases, the similarity between a foreign antigen and a host protein is usually incomplete. A protein can offer many different regions as suitable targets for an immunological attack. The diversified immune system is an instrument with many strings. From the point of view of the species, the black holes offer no difficulties. The individual is exchangeable—the species covers all its black holes through the vast polymorphism of the MHC system.

Autoimmune Diseases

How reliable is the tolerance against "self" proteins? It is surprisingly high, although not absolute. An organism cannot always avoid reacting against its own tissues. If such reactions become intense, they can lead to autoimmune diseases. Lupus, a serious disease of skin and internal organisms, rheumatoid arthritis, and certain disorders of the thyroid and adrenal glands are among the most well known examples. Other skin diseases, kidney inflammations, diabetes, multiple sclerosis, and other diseases of the central nervous system are also suspected to have autoimmune components. Here you enter the backyard of the MHC system. Some autoimmune diseases are more common in people with certain MHC types than in others. The strongest connection is between the MHC type B27 and a severe joint disease called ankylosing spondylitis, a severe arthritis of the spine. Not all B27-positive people develop this painful and incapacitating disease, but practically all who do develop it are B27-positive. According to one hypothesis, the B27 protein may bind bacterial or other antigens that closely resemble some normal host proteins.[3] Presentation of the foreign antigen to the immune system may elicit an autoimmune reaction that attacks the skeleton and particularly the joints more aggressively than other tissues. This is presumably not due to the breakdown of natural tolerance to "self" MHC components, but rather to the special ability of a certain MHC variant to bind a widely prevalent foreign antigen. This binding would not be limited to cells of the immune system. Tight binding of the antigen to B27 in some of the normal solid tissues would provide a target for autoimmune reactions that attack the skeleton. Even if the system were to function perfectly, it is open to "accidents" of this or similar types. This is hardly surprising. On the contrary, it is astounding that mistakes do not occur more often.

Autoimmune diseases can therefore be elicited in at least two ways: either through an excessively tight binding of a foreign antigen to a particular MHC molecule that may affect cells of the immune system and of solid tissue, or through incomplete tolerance to "self" antigens, due to some defect in the normal process whereby "self-reactive" T-cells are eliminated.

Graft Rejection Revisited

After this survey of our current view of the MHC system, let us now return to its experimental and conceptual origins, the rejection of foreign grafts. What is this reaction due to, and does it have any relevance to the normal organism?

The answer to the first question is not yet in, but there are two competing hypotheses. According to the first, the T-cell system recognizes a foreign MHC molecule because it isn't exactly identical to its own molecules. T-cells with the corresponding, complementary receptor respond to the distinctive features of the foreign MHC molecule, different from self-MHC. Even a single "point mutation," the substitution of one amino acid in a normal host MHC protein for a different amino acid, is sufficient to bring about a full-blown rejection reaction. The second hypothesis proposes that the foreign MHC molecule is not antigenic for the host as such, but only after it has, like all other antigens, been broken down by macrophages followed by the presentation of its breakdown products to the T-cells. However, neither explanation can explain all available facts, and the issue is still unsolved.

The rejection reaction against foreign cells has little significance in any context other than the transfer of cells between individuals. Blood transfusion is one example. Rejection of the foreign lymphocytes is important, because it might otherwise cause a similar damage as in immunologically compromised bone-marrow transplant recipients. But blood transfusion is a medical intervention. Sexual intercourse is the most natural form of cellular transfer. The sperms are protected against rejection, but other cells of the ejaculate, including lymphocytes, are rejected just like transfused white blood cells. The rejection of fetal cells that have made their way into the mother's circulation may be of major importance. The placental cells of the fetus have to establish a foothold in the uterine wall. They have a considerable capacity to invade tissues. Now and then they can even be found in the lung capillaries of pregnant women. They can look quite dangerous, as they seem to be trying to invade the lung tissue just like cancer cells might do. But this does not happen. The placenta must normally allow the "invasion" of the maternal uterine wall, but in the lung the misplaced cells are eliminated by the rejection reaction.

The Female Mouse Chooses Her Mate through an "MHC-type" Typing with the Help of Her Sense of Smell

The reader may think that this is a joke, but it is not. In one experiment, performed for an entirely unrelated purpose, groups of three mice, one male and two females, were put into a number of cages. The aim was to produce offspring of the male's inbred strain and also F_1-hybrid mice between his strain and a foreign strain. One female belonged to the same strain as the male, whereas the other was from a foreign strain. The results of matings in mice can be be determined very quickly through detection of the so-called vaginal plugs. Surprisingly, it was found that the male mated with the female from the foreign strain considerably more often than with the female from his own strain. But upon closer study, it was determined that this choice depended on female rather than on male preference. In a more sophisticated experimental system, females were placed at the far end of a Y-shaped cage. Layers of sawdust bedding impregnated with the urine of two different males were placed in the arms of the Y. One sample came from a male of the same strain as the female, the other from a male of a foreign strain. The females were in heat. Which branch of the Y would the female choose? Most of the time, she went in the direction of the urine from the male of the foreign strain.

It was also found that the presence of a foreign male or the smell of a foreign male's urine can even affect a fertilized female. If such a female had mated with a male from her own strain, exposure to the secretions of a foreign male could induce an abortion before the egg had a chance to implant into the uterus.

This experiment doesn't prove that the female chooses the foreign male on the basis of his MHC type. But that is exactly what she does. This was demonstrated with the help of a so-called congenic mouse strain that had been produced earlier by the father of transplantation immunology, George Snell. Congenic strains are genetically identical, but they have *different* MHC markers. Snell started with an ordinary F_1 crossing between two strains, A and B, carrying different MHC markers. He back-crossed the AB hybrids to the A strain and typed the offspring for MHC. He selected the offspring that carried the MHC of the B strain and crossed them again with the A strain. He continued with back crossings to A while selecting for retention of the B strain's MHC for about ten generations. Gradually, a congenic state is reached: two strains that are genetically identical except for the MHC genes that had been selectively retained from the B strain. There are now a great number of congenic strains available for studies on MHC. When female mice were given the choice of males from their own strain or from a congenic strain, identical for all genes except for their MHC, the females selected the foreign MHC males for mating. The smell of the urine of the foreign male was sufficient for this choice.

Are there similar mechanisms for sexual preference in other mammals? Does human body odor also vary, depending on our MHC? Nothing is known about that, but it is interesting to note that trained dogs identify individual humans depending on their unique body odor. They make no mistakes. But they cannot distinguish between identical twins, nor do they want to. Attempts have been made to train experienced police dogs to distinguish between identical twins through the use of a variety of perfumes, soaps, or other artificial scents. But the police dogs refused to distinguish between twins. Their identification was determined by the body odor and could not be changed by cosmetics. There is no evidence that the MHC antigen itself is responsible for the ability of the dogs to distinguish between unrelated individuals, but the experiments with mice are at least consistent with that possibility.

Sexual selection is a powerful evolutionary instrument. If females prefer males with foreign MHC markers to those with identical MHC types, they contribute to the maintenance of the MHC diversity in the species. But what does the female's sense of smell actually recognize? Is it the MHC proteins or their degradation products that determine the smell? That possibility cannot be excluded, but it is highly unlikely. As has probably become evident from earlier sections of this chapter, the MHC molecules play a major role in immune recognition. It is also known, however, that the large MHC gene complex contains genes involved in other processes. It is therefore likely that the mixture of odoriferous substances in the urine is slightly—but for the mouse olfactory system, perceptibly—different, depending on the exact constellation of the MHC genes in a given animal. Whatever the explanation, these experiments contribute to the already strong impression that MHC diversity is maintained by powerful selective mechanisms. Such mechanisms may have evolved because of the protective value of MHC polymorphism against major epidemics at the level of the entire species, as discussed earlier.

Epilogue: The Seventh Seal

Ingmar Bergman has turned seventy. His great films are shown during the festival week, and I am watching *The Seventh Seal* for the second time. Almost four decade have passed since I first saw it. I find to my surprise that it has lived in my memory all this time, even though I wasn't aware of it. I know the dialogue, the changes of scenery, the images—I sense them coming before I see them on the screen. The plague is ravaging medieval Sweden. The stern lord, Death, has a great deal to do. And yet he has time to play chess with the knight. The knight loses the game and must join the final "danse macabre." Death drags him away together with his traveling companions, all of whom happened to be gathering in the great castle. Each of them represents an entire world unto himself. We are able to peer into their innermost beings during the few moments that Bergman's camera is focused on them. But all these individual worlds are erased when the silhouettes pass by, trailing after the figure of Death on the mountain ridge, in front of the frightened but happy young jester couple and their little son who were saved by the knight during his self-sacrificing game of chess with Death.

The unforgettable performance of Anders Ek in the role of the flagellant priest has been etched indelibly onto my memory more than anything else in the film. Ignorant about the plague bacterium and immunological defenses, the flagellants drag themselves on, dishevelled, half naked, sick and crippled, as they whip themselves and each other with all conceivable instruments before the horrified villagers. The priest showers the still healthy onlookers with insulting and taunting words, warning them that they should not think that their stupid, bloated, and self-righteous indifference or that the beauty and strength of the young will last more than a week or so more, perhaps even only a few days or a few hours. The thesis that prompts the words and deeds of the flagellants and the priest is so clear that it needs no further explanation: the plague is God's rightful punishment for man's sinful life. Only through the mortification of the flesh can they hope to drive out sin.

Yes, sin, with sexuality at its center, is the fundamental thesis. But sexuality is one of evolution's most powerful instruments. The biological battle between the plague bacterium, rats, and humans was completely hidden from the medieval sight, but it was precisely this battle that became the determining factor. All three species were walking a tightrope. Genetic variability and recombination within the two mammalian species had led to their victory and to the defeat of the plague bacterium, at least in its virulent form.

In an idyllic morning scene in the film, the visionary jester-juggler gazes at his little son and tells his young wife and companion that the boy "will surpass us as an artist. I can juggle two, maybe three or even more balls at the same time, but he'll be able to do more. He'll be able to make a ball stop in mid-air!"

No, he'll never be able to do that. All his eventual achievements, all experimentation will have to stay within the limits of natural law. The same is true for the eternal game of the genes. But genes make use of all possible mechanisms permitted by their structure to create new variants. The plague bacterium operates blindly, as do all other organisms, but no more or less blindly than humans who consider themselves so much more rational, conscious, and willful. Both are driven by the same goal—the "blind will" of DNA to reproduce itself.[4] The game of gene variation does not know "what it wants," but it does provide the means to deal with new and changed situations. If we view the game from a narrow human point of view, we are likely to look on the variants as good or bad, threatening or benign. But the bacterium does not care about us. Our very closely related cousins, the rats, and we ourselves, must constantly strengthen and broaden our immunological defenses to enable us to cope with new variants that the bacterium is able to produce to escape our immune defenses. In the long run, the DNA game works for the survival of all three species. A passenger in the sleeping compartment of a train who is disturbed by the clattering noise and blows up the compartment to stop it will not travel very far. Similarly, to ensure its own survival, the bacterium must find a suitable balance between reproducing itself too much, with fatal consequences for both itself and its host, and reproducing too little, with the resulting danger that it may be weeded out. It competes not only with its hosts and their effective immunological systems, but also with other bacteria, including its own well-adapted and harmless cousins in the normal mammalian intestinal flora. Its competitive power is based on the DNA game. Most bacteria reproduce their own type faithfully on most cell divisions, but new variants are continuously generated in their large populations, ready to try their luck in the universal competition among different kinds of bacteria and also within the population of their own kind. The DNA of the bacteria mutate by similar mechanisms as the DNA of higher organisms. It is basically the same Monte Carlo game, but it does differ in many details. The bacteria contain an entire world of even smaller microorganisms, the bacterial viruses and other "self-replicating genetic elements" that "earn their livelihood" by parasitizing bacterial cells just as bacteria parasitize mammals. Some bacterial viruses provide their bacterial hosts with entirely new characteristics. They function just like the cell's own genes. Even the sexuality of the bacteria, the ability of a "male" bacterium to transfer its DNA to a recipient "female" through a microscopically detectable sexual act, called conjugation, is determined by a viruslike segment of DNA called the F-particle. Bacterial cells infected with such an F-particle become males while their uninfected counterparts function as females. If a bacterial cell is "cured" of its F-particle by antibiotic therapy, it changes sex. Sexual reproduction is not mandatory and not even very important for bacteria. They may experiment with it, but they have many other and considerably faster methods that allow them to recombine or otherwise change their genetic material. Among them, the "jumping genes" or transposons are perhaps the most remarkable. They resemble bacterial viruses in many ways. They can move from one region of a chromosome to another, and may activate or inactivate adjacent genes in the course of the process. It is conceivable that the transposons had been derived from bacterial viruses that have placed themselves in the service of their host bacterial cell to secure their own survival. According to a different alternative, they have evolved from the genes of the bacterial cell itself. Activation of some transposons may endanger the host organism, if it leads to the production of toxins, or makes the bacterium resistant to antibiotics. But it can also produce beneficial effects, expressed in a milder course of an infectious disease.

DNA Is the Raw Material of Evolution, Variation Is Its Most Important Survival Instrument, Selection Provides Its Implementation Principle

The same basic principles regulate the evolution of the plague bacterium and its two highly developed hosts, rats and humans. From the perspective of the bacterium, the two mammalian species are just about equally high. Differences between them must appear relatively insignificant from the bacteria's point of view. Unlike the bacteria, however, the mammalian hosts do not have the capacity to vary their genetic material with comparable speed. Their experimentation is more complicated and farsighted, but no less inventive. As I have described elsewhere,[5] the great triumph of sexuality in all the higher plants and animals may be at least partly due to its chromosome stabilizing effect, an insurance against excessive gene rearrangements. Only cells with relatively stable genetic material can pass through the eye of a needle, the precise reduction division of germ cells, a requirement for sexual reproduction. But how can the relatively stable world of higher vertebrates cope with the unbelievable flexibility of microorganisms? What obstacles can it place in the way of the perpetual game played by creatures with such a rapid reproduction?

The MHC system, in combination with the diversity of the immunoglobulin (Ig) and the TCR genes, provides the most important barriers. Even the most clever bacterium can punch only a few holes in the compact protection provided by the large gene pool of the entire human species. The black death in *The Seventh Seal* could have made only a few holes in this defense barrier, like the epidemics that killed 60 percent of the people in the Dutch immigrant colony in Surinam. The total MHC, Ig, and TCR repertoire of the species could wipe out the black death and convert that immense tragedy into a few transient footsteps in the sand. But what would happen if a virus were to wipe out the entire immune system? What is happening with the curse of our own time, AIDS? We will examine that question in the next chapter.

8

AIDS

Catastrophe and Euphoria at the World Congress on AIDS in Stockholm, 1988

Almost 7,000 participants filled the light and spacious meeting areas of the Älvsjö conference center during the great world congress on AIDS in Stockholm in June 1988. The entire week-long meeting dealt with only one virus, HIV, but there were twice as many participants as at the large international congresses that deal with all viruses. At an ordinary virology meeting, half a day would have been devoted to AIDS, and the session would have run in parallel with a dozen other sessions dealing with other viruses.

There was a peculiar atmosphere of cheerfulness, almost euphoria, so obviously different from the mood that usually prevails at large international meetings. Most large congresses lack the intensity of the small and scientifically more rewarding symposia. Sometimes they are merely social gatherings with a scientific pretext, but they also lack the festive mood of more overtly social events. They tend to be hybrids between scientific exchange and pleasant social activity—and fail at both. At this meeting, the atmosphere was entirely different. I could already sense this the first morning, and my impression was strengthened during the week. At first I thought this was due to the unusually efficient organization of the meeting, but I later realized that although this was one of the reasons, it was not the main factor.

The AIDS epidemic is a growing catastrophe. It is the worst biological disaster to befall our species in modern times. It is sometimes compared with the plague, and there are certainly

some parallels. But if so, how is it possible to explain the enthusiastic atmosphere of the meeting? What is the crucial difference
between the participants at the AIDS congress and the reactions
of socially responsible people to large epidemics in the past?

I found several possible answers—or, more precisely, probable
contibuting factors—as the week went by. We now have modern
science at our disposal. Molecular biology is precise and potentially powerful. The strident minorities within our culture who
blame science for many of the ills of society, including the
deterioration of the environment and the proliferation of nuclear
weapons, and who see molecular biology as a threat to the
freedom and integrity of humanity, do not realize that the rapid
identification of HIV, only three years after the start of the
epidemic, was achieved by that very science.

During the short time that has elapsed since the discovery of
the AIDS virus, new discoveries have already become not only
accepted but even "classical" knowledge. I tried to pick up the
mood of the discussions in the lecture halls and, more important,
the tone of conversations held in the corridors and during coffee
breaks.

All felt that they were in the same boat. The situation was
ominous, but not hopeless. There certainly was a great deal of
competition among, and sometimes even within, the various
research groups, but in that regard this was no different than
other scientific fields. Societal pressures and the scientists' desire
to solve the problem—or at least to contribute to its solution—
were more compelling and urgent than in any other field. But I
had a strong feeling that other factors may have contributed to
the optimistic atmosphere as well.

The congress was a living demonstration of the contention that
the AIDS problem affects all aspects of human relations. Gathered there under one roof were representatives of many tradition-
ally quite distant disciplines. The molecular biologists were obviously leading the scientific development. They commanded the
greatest respect and drew the largest audiences. The students
looked at them in the way that teenagers tend to regard fighter
pilots in countries at war.

Classical virologists were more sparsely represented. This was
understandable, because the identification of the AIDS virus had

been accomplished. Many important goals remained for the virologists, but they were of more peripheral interest to the majority of the AIDS scientific community. The search for HIV-related nonhuman viruses that could provide an authentic model for AIDS appeared to be the most important.

There was some pessimism among the immunologists who originally defined AIDS as the breakdown of the immune system. Many unexpected problems have arisen in relation to their obvious goal—vaccination against HIV. It turned out that HIV-infected people can mount a strong immune response against the virus and virus-infected cells, but they nevertheless develop the disease. The killer cells described in the previous chapter can destroy HIV-infected cells in the test tube quite effectively, at least during the initial, symptom-free stages of the infection. Similar immune responses can easily conquer other viral infections, including those caused by other members of the retrovirus family, to which HIV belongs. But HIV is evasive. It finds a sanctuary, a lair deeply buried in the interior of several cell types, including cells of the immune system itself. It hides largely but not exclusively in the helper T-cells. The immune breakdown is associated with the disappearance of the helper cells.

It is doubtful that the immune system can be mobilized to fight this attack from within because the infection has converted the protector, the "policeman," into an assailant. There is still the hope that a vaccine might work at the very earliest stages of infection, immediately after entry of the virus into the body, before it has had a chance to find its niche. Conventional vaccination cannot reach the virus after this stage, although immunological support measures might be useful in combination with other treatments. We will return to this point.

The epidemiologists played an important role as the messengers of reality. They traced the virus's strange journey through our two most important body fluids, blood and sperm, through towns and villages, through underdeveloped and industrialized nations, between homosexuals and heterosexuals, among drug addicts, hemophilia patients, and other recipients of blood transfusions. They described with the same detachment the passage of the virus between unsuspecting young lovers or married couples and from the mother to her newborn child. Uncounted numbers of human tragedies followed apparently trivial exposures such as a single casual sexual contact or an ordinary blood transfusion. The merciless rampage of the virus several years later makes Greek tragedies seem mere bagatelles by comparison. The cold statistics of the epidemiological reports looked threatening. Nevertheless, there were gratifying signs that the statistics were having an effect on the behavior of some of the major risk groups. In the large American cities where the epidemic started, homosexuals have now apparently modified their behavior, as reflected by a decrease in the number of new infections.

The sexual freedom that followed the advent of the birth control pill has obviously been severely shaken. The information campaigns against AIDS have made progress, and have even led to a remarkable revival in the previously threatened condom industry. But nobody can tell whether information will maintain its impact over longer periods of time. At the congress, lectures by epidemiologists attracted large audiences who listened with breathless intensity. It reminded me of the times I listened surreptitiously to the BBC during the German occupation. Then, like now, the audience was anxious to learn the truth about the situation, free of politically colored propaganda, emotional exaggerations, and disparaging denials.

Some of the more mathematically oriented epidemiologists were not content with merely reporting the newest statistical information on the regional distribution of the epidemic and the risk groups. They tried to look into the future and predict the epidemic's course. Their uniformly dismal sermons were met with shock, silence, and all shades of skepticism and denial. Both in private discussions and in newspaper interviews, the critics eagerly attacked details of the reports to cast doubt on their general conclusions. Had it not been predicted that the frequency of HIV infection in risk-group C in city A would increase at X percent during the upcoming six months? The frequency had in fact not increased—the epidemiologists were wrong and their grim prognoses therefore could not be trusted. I had a strong sense of déjà vu—isn't this exactly the language of wishful thinking?

At the same time, it was also obvious that it could have been much worse. HIV is a deadly virus, but it is not highly infectious.

That's our bit of good luck in the midst of misfortune. This was evident from the many studies of couples in which one partner was known to be infected with HIV.[1] There were considerable quantitative differences between these reports. The frequency of virus transmission to the unprotected sexual partner varied widely from 10 percent to 86 percent, depending on country and ethnic group, and it was possible to identify certain factors that affected this risk. Simultaneous infection with other sexually transmitted diseases also increased the risk of HIV transmission. Sores on the genitals and absence of circumcision were additional risk factors. The likelihood of transmission of the virus to a partner was increased when the infected person began to show symptoms of AIDS. This is understandable, because breakdown of the immune system promotes continuous replication of the virus in the body, and the likelihood of infection increases with increasing amounts of virus. From studies with other and better understood animal retroviruses, we also know that susceptibility to infection can vary genetically. Differences in the susceptibility of host cells to virus penetration and replication and the ability of the host to respond promptly to the first virus infection are dependent, among other things, on the variations of the MHC system within the species (see the chapter on "Biological Individuality"). In the case of HIV, no information is yet available on such genetic factors, but this probably only reflects the fact that humans are much more difficult to study from the genetic point of view than inbred mice. Nevertheless, there is no doubt that genetic differences can affect the susceptibility to infection with HIV or even the development of the disease.

The sociologists of sexuality played an important role at the congress, even though they seemed like dignitaries from an exotic land. The largely medical-biological audiences responded with a mixture of interest and skepticism. Is this science, is it really relevant? But every now and then sudden, liberating laughter would burst forth, usually in response to the provocatively free descriptions of sexual behavior presented with brilliant eloquence by the erudite humanists. They had a strong sense of humor—macabre, urbanized or rather metropolitan, verging on the cynical but with an undertone of warmth and humane understanding. They confirmed the feeling that we were all in the same boat—

but a bigger vessel than the AIDS boat by itself. Sexuality is one of our primal urges, whether we like it or not. It interests us all—we might as well stop being hypocritical about it. It was a relief for the audience to hear it spelled out so explicitly. But the description of the sexual landscape also had an opposite, darker side: misunderstanding, cruelty, oppression, discrimination, exploitation, and a wasteland of irreparable psychological harm. The black or white, "good guy/bad guy" stereotypes of pioneer America were reflected by the expression "homophobia," the heterosexuals' dread of homosexuals, and the equivalent madness of "gay identity" that homophobia released among homosexuals. The victims and the perpetrators of discrimination are bound together by a subconscious and inexorable logic.

According to the experts, human sexual behavior has not been adequately studied, in spite of the Kinsey Report and other studies that were often based on dubious methods of data collection and contained relatively antiquated information. The foremost scientific representative of the field at the congress, John Gagnon, also criticized the tendency of AIDS researchers to discuss sexuality in relation to AIDS rather than to analyze the AIDS epidemic from a solid background of knowledge of human sexuality.[2] In his words,

Much of the most important work that has been conducted on sexuality, from Freud to Kinsey to Foucault, has been an attempt to understand the way sexuality was intertwined with the rest of social, cultural and psychological life. The key words are *to understand*. Most of the current interest in sexuality is motivated nearly entirely by the urgent need to keep people alive in the face of the epidemic. . . . The sexual questions that are posed, of all the questions that could be asked, are generated by a concern for the transmission of HIV. . . . A strong consequence of this disease focus is that *sex itself can become confused with disease and being sexual in various ways becomes treated as an illness or as evidence of illness.* Sexuality is a form of conduct that is complexly related to pleasure, sin, reproduction, getting old, growing up, enduring loss, and the like. . . . The ways in which we change our conduct to limit transmission will have an impact of the purposes of sex in the larger society. . . . Most immediately, science about sex is news, AIDS is news, and the news about sex and AIDS affects those who read or hear or see it as well as those who make policy about it.

Even within the constraints of a concern for AIDS, a narrow view of sexual behavior may be effective if all that we are concerned with is social bookkeeping and epidemiological modeling, but it will be inadequate to the task of understanding behavior in a way that results in behavior change. Sexual conduct is embedded in culture and in social relations—as we begin to deal with this dimension of the spread of HIV and the resultant disease processes, we will need to know more than how old, how often, when, and with whom—we will need to know a great deal more about why.

There were many other professional groups attending the congress: physicians who care for AIDS patients, sex educators who design informational programs, youth advisors, members of voluntary organizations that care for the sick and dying, and even AIDS patients themselves, who had been provided a special resting room in the congress hall. They did not give any talks, but they were present and they listened. Did they come to the meetings out of hope or fear? Were they there to emphasize their urgency and the desperation of their plight? Were they driven by the same interest that a victim might show for his assailant, did they wish to confront the incomprehensible virus that had undermined the strong wall that had protected them so unobtrusively against the outside world in the past? Did they wish to understand how so many harmless microorganisms living in the human digestive tract, on our skin, in our body apertures, and in our environment could fly into such a rage and transform themselves into destructive, wild beasts? Or did they want to warn us about the road we risk traveling if we were to follow in their footsteps? All of these—any of these?

Large quilts covered the walls of the plenary hall. Names were sewn on them: Johnny, Dick, Tommy. One last tribute to a dead friend. But no noticeable sense of sorrow pervaded the congress. Or had the sorrow merely changed its expression? Had it turned white as among the Buddhists—was the mortal threat countered with a euphoric will to live? Had the sorrow been replaced by an experience of true solidarity that could transgress political and disciplinary barriers and convey a sense of meaning to all scientific and other activities in this field—a sense of purpose that is lacking in many other contexts?

The Virus and Its Rampage

How have we gotten to this point? Where did the virus originate, how could it suddenly come crashing down on an unsuspecting world at the end of the 1970s?

It is likely that HIV was a relatively isolated virus, limited to small, poor, and undernourished groups of people among whom high mortality was taken for granted and where different causes of death were not accurately determined, before it suddenly spread all over the world through vastly increased international contacts. There is no rational alternative to this explanation. Many irrational ideas have been proposed in a number of contexts. These can best be looked upon as fantasies with heavy political or mythological overtones. One such "political" theory has been proposed by an East German scientist who claimed that the virus might have escaped from an American military research institution working on the development of biological weapons. The theory has gained acceptance in several of the former East Bloc countries and even among some sympathizers in the West despite its obvious absurdity. Another myth, created by some confused environmentalists, suggested that AIDS might have appeared as a result of the pollution of nature by humans. Notions of this type have their roots in age-old concepts of divine retribution for sin as the cause of plagues and epidemics. It is not surprising that some religious groups have propounded the idea that AIDS is God's punishment for a sinful life.

The entire spectrum of human dreams, hopes, aggressions, guilt feelings, and apprehensions are expressed in these fantasies. They remind me of other irrational phenomena such as astrology—the absurd belief that momentary spatial relationships of cold and indifferent stars, positioned in outer space by physical forces during the month of birth, can be used to predict a person's characteristics over a lifetime. Reports that even modern military commanders or politicians use this method to predict the chances of a crucial battle or competition indicates that our overall rationality has not progressed very far since Roman commanders predicted their immediate future by examining the intestines of chickens. It is remarkable that such habits survive even in our time, in spite of our scientific development. It is startling that otherwise rational people can yield so easily to the temptation to see a connection between independent phenomena that happened to coincide in time.

A virus is no mythological creature. It is not generated from nothing or from inorganic matter. Its strategy requires no supernatural explanation. All viruses have an organic structure built according to genetic instructions that followed the same basic principles as your body or mine. Viruses use the same genetic code language as our own DNA. They find their way in and out of our cells like old dogs who know the smells in every corner of the house. They subvert and use the machinery of the cell for their own purposes, and can proceed in different ways: gently like a polite guest, or destructively like a gang of vandals. What they do and why and when they do it is determined by their own genetic information, a finely polished product of evolution after many millions of years of selection. The interaction of viruses with cells occurs with a precision that makes our most sophisticated modern instruments seem no more than awkward stone-age tools. We will examine this interaction more closely, but first let's take a short look at history.

Our concepts of viruses have changed radically over the course of time. Use of the Latin word *virus*, meaning poison, dates back to a time before it was known whether they represented chemical poisons or living organisms. They were first called "filterable viruses," because their capacity to produce disease was unchanged after the infectious matter was passed through filters with pores small enough to trap the larger, microscopically visible bacteria. But it became obvious that biological organisms were involved when it was found that the activity of the viruses increased after they were passed through sensitive host animals, fertilized chicken eggs, and later, tissue culture. The virus-infected cells often became sick and died. The microscopic features of their death battle differed, depending on the virus. After the development of the electron microscope, the previously invisible virus particles became physical realities appearing in multiple geometric forms and with remarkable beauty. It also became clear that viruses were cellular parasites. In contrast to bacteria and other independent microorganisms, viruses can reproduce only inside other cells and never in the free form.

Serum from patients who recovered from a viral infection was often able to neutralize or interfere with the ability of corresponding or similar viruses to infect cells in tissue culture. Many of our modern methods of virus diagnosis and the identification of different subtypes of a single virus family are based on "serum neutralization reactions" or similar reactions in which an identifiable "flag," a dye molecule or a radioactive isotope, is attached to the antibody to allow detection of binding to virus-infected cells.

The discovery that virus replication in tissue culture is accompanied by microscopically observable pathological changes in the cells opened the door to the development of vaccines against polio and many other diseases. Virus growth in tissue culture also led to the identification of many previously unknown viruses in normal human tissues that were not known to be associated with any disease. In the mid-1950s, a symposium entitled "Viruses in Search of a Disease" was held in New York. The title is an allusion to the play "Six Characters in Search of an Author" by Luigi Pirandello and is an interesting reflection of a historical misconception. Viruses were first identified as agents that cause disease, but the notion that every virus must have its own disease became more and more unrealistic during the ensuing years. Like all other living creatures, each virus had been selected for survival, for the most effective transmission of its genes from cell to cell, from host organism to host organism. If a virus produces illness in a host, it reduces its own chances for survival. Many viruses have developed special mechanisms that allow them to become "latent" for the entire lifetime of the whole organism without causing much or any trouble.[3] Disease-causing viruses are the rare exception among viruses. They are like mad dogs or frenzied sharks that attack people bathing at the beach.

HIV belongs to the family of viruses known as lentiviruses, a subclass of the larger group of retroviruses. There are two clearly defined human lentiviruses, HIV-1 and HIV-2. Other closely related lentiviruses have chosen monkeys as their natural hosts. The difference between HIV-1 and HIV-2 is greater than that between HIV-2 and one of the monkey viruses. These kinds of virus families are very common; their shared traits are called "conserved." A characteristic trait of the HIV family is the ability to infect one of the most important players of the "immunological orchestra," the helper T-cell, often referred to as the T-4 cells. T-4 cells have a characteristic membrane component, a protein called CD4. HIV-1 and HIV-2 and the counterpart monkey viruses have "chosen" to interact with the CD4 molecule during the first step of the infectious process. CD4 serves as the cell's receptor for HIV. The virus particle that binds to the receptor will penetrate and initiate its life cycle inside the cell.

The total breakdown of the helper T-cells constitutes the most characteristic feature of AIDS. Among the HIV-like viruses of apes, there are some virus variants that also affect the T-4 cells, but that do not cause any AIDS-like illness. Neither does the human HIV virus induce any serious disease in chimpanzees, despite the fact that this closely related evolutionary cousin of ours is infected in exactly the same way as humans. The penetration of the virus into helper T-cells is therefore a necessary but not sufficient condition for the development of AIDS.

We don't know whether the two disease-causing variants HIV-1 and HIV-2 have existed in their present form before the onset of the worldwide epidemic, or if they have recently developed through mutation from harmless ancestors. HIV-1 and HIV-2 share only 40 percent of their genetic material with each other, and it is unlikely that two such different variants would simultaneously have been converted from harmless to disease-causing viruses. It is also unlikely that both variants would have "jumped" from apes to humans at the same time, although this is possible for HIV-2, the more monkeylike of the two viruses. It is more likely that HIV-1 and HIV-2 and other, as yet unidentified HIV variants have been around long before our time, carried by isolated human societies living under difficult conditions and among whom starvation, poverty, parasitic disease, war, and other kinds of social disruption cause a high mortality rate. A short average life span is one of the givens in these cultures, in which underdeveloped medical systems are unable to determine causes of death more effectively. Previously unknown diseases can easily pass through these societies without being noticed.

The best bit of good fortune, if one can speak of "fortune" in connection with the AIDS catastrophe, concerns the extremely restricted ability of the virus to spread. As we know, it is transmitted by body fluids, mainly blood and semen. Had it been transmitted by water, air, foodstuffs, or casual contacts, as are so many other viruses, we would have witnessed a global catastrophe of far greater dimensions.

Many other retroviruses have been recognized long before HIV. They have been found in chickens, mice, cats, apes, cows, sheep, horses and, much less frequently, in humans. Most of them are completely harmless, but some can cause leukemia or breast cancer, provided that they infect a genetically susceptible host animal in whose cells they can replicate.[4] Such animals are often rare genetic variants, selected by the investigator for study. However, in nature most animals are genetically resistant and can keep even these viruses under control with the help of their immune systems.

But why does HIV cause the immune system to collapse? What is the essential difference between HIV and its more benign relatives? Is it only a question of the degree of immune impairment? It is known that some mouse leukemia viruses can inhibit the immune system to a certain extent, even though they might not produce as complete a breakdown as HIV-1 does in AIDS. However, cat (feline) leukemia virus (FELV) has certain effects whose clinical manifestations are reminiscent of AIDS. FELV is transmitted among cats like an ordinary infectious disease, but while the risk that a virus-infected animal will develop leukemia is only 5-10 percent, some of the infected cats die of an inflammation of the peritoneum called infectious peritonitis. This occurs when the immune system is damaged by the virus to such an extent that the normal intestinal bacteria break through the protective barrier of the lymphoid system and produce a generalized sepsis. It was no coincidence that investigators of cat leukemia were among the first to suspect that the AIDS virus might be a member of the retrovirus family. It is also no coincidence that the two scientists who first isolated HIV, Luc Montagnier in Paris and Robert Gallo in the United States, had previously worked with other retroviruses. Gallo had, among other things, isolated HTLV-1, the only known leukemia virus of humans that causes a rare form of adult T-cell leukemia, which occurs mostly in southern Japan and in the Caribbean. Without these previous advances in the retrovirus field, we would certainly still be ignorant about the origin and nature of AIDS.

The Molecular Strategy of HIV and Potential Therapeutic Targets

The astounding fact that we know so much about the retrovirus family stems from a series of lucky coincidences. The following seemingly unconnected factors have been instrumental in this connection.

During the time of President Kennedy, a man traveled to the moon. The goal of the Apollo project was meaningless in itself, and began primarily as a result of political pressures related to the maintenance of national prestige in the Cold War with the Soviet Union. But the development of computer technology was a very significant by-product of the Apollo project. President Nixon wanted to do something even more important when he took the initiative with "The Cancer Act," a piece of legislation that provided increased support for cancer research. At that time, many believed that most human cancers were caused by viruses.[5] The huge investment of resources didn't lead to the desired result, because the most important human tumors are not caused by viruses. However, the Nixon project accelerated the development of modern molecular biology, and it heavily promoted the kind of research on retroviruses that was to become so important when the global endemic of AIDS struck a decade later.

Retroviruses, originally called RNA tumor viruses, go in and out of the cell's chromosomes. Their genetic information is written in the form of DNA as long as they remain integrated with the chromosome in this "proviral" form. In the next phase, when the virus is scheduled to undergo replication and move on to a new cell, it converts or "transcribes" its DNA into RNA. The viral RNA provides instructions to the cell's protein-synthesizing machinery to produce viral proteins, the building blocks of the virus, in addition to or instead of cellular proteins. The newly produced viral proteins wrap themselves around the viral RNA and assemble into virus particles, after which they are released from the cell. They must then find a new target cell that can bind the virus and allow it to replicate or to continue its existence in a latent form. The virus particles bind only to cells that contain the membrane component that acts as the cell's special "antenna" to "receive" the virus. HIV has chosen to attach itself to the CD4 molecule on the membrane of the helper T-cells. Other retroviruses have chosen different receptor molecules and other cells. This choice represents one of several factors that determine which cells can be infected by a given retrovirus. When the virus has entered its new host cell, its genetic information is again rewritten from RNA to DNA, after which the DNA (proviral) copy plants itself among the genes of the cell. This shuttling between the RNA and DNA forms of the viral genetic information is a distinctive characteristic of retroviruses.

HIV is an unusual retrovirus. Like other retroviruses, it has three major genes, but it also has a remarkable collection of minor genes, which we shall examine in more detail. One of the three major genes, called *gag*, is responsible for the production of the inner viral protein, the so-called capsid protein, which gives the viral particle its basic structure and protects the viral RNA from degradation. The other major large gene, *env*, carries the blueprint for the viral envelope. If one compares the capsid protein to the skin that protects our internal tissues, the envelope can be likened to our clothing or, rather, to a warm coat that protects us from harsh winds. In fact, it protects the virus particle against destruction in the circulation and in a variety of body fluids. The proteins of the envelope are also responsible for the capacity of the virus to bind to the correct target cell, as described above. In the case of HIV, the *env* protein fits into the helper T-cell's CD4 receptor molecule like a key fits into a lock.

The third major gene, *pol*, produces an enzyme that has given the retrovirus family its name. It is found only in retroviruses and is a prerequisite for the viral life cycle. It transcribes RNA into DNA in a "reverse" direction, so called because the usual cellular enzymes and also other viral enzymes transcribe in the other direction, from DNA into RNA. Consequently, it is called "reverse transcriptase" and is the basis for the name "retrovirus."

After the virus has become bound to the CD4 receptor on the target cell, the viral envelope fuses with the cellular membrane. This doesn't cause any problems because the biochemical composition of the viral envelope is very similar to that of the cell membrane. The viral RNA is thereafter transported to the inner part of the cell, where it drops out of the virus particle like the seed from cut-up fruit.

The virus uses the cell's protein-degrading enzymes to liberate the RNA from the capsid proteins, but the liberated RNA doesn't remain in the form of free RNA for long. The reverse transcriptase, brought into the cell as a part of the virus, immediately begins to transcribe the RNA into DNA. The newly produced copy of proviral DNA is then integrated among the cellular genes. Contrary to other types of viruses, the retroviral DNA doesn't take command of the cell's protein synthesis, which adapts smoothly to the normal processes of cell growth and cell division. The presence of the viral DNA doesn't disturb the life of the cell. It replicates together with the cellular DNA prior to the next cell division and behaves in every respect like ordinary cellular genes. But it also preserves its special proviral status. It can be activated to transcribe its own DNA-encoded instructions into RNA again so that new virus proteins can be produced and assemble into new virus particles, as already mentioned. When the cell becomes senescent or is exposed to toxins, the virus may behave like a pilot who ejects himself from a damaged airplane. In lymphocytes, the virus can even be activated by the cell's normal reaction against antigens associated with other viral or bacterial infections. This is especially important for HIV-infected people who are still healthy. Chance infections can activate their HIV with virus production and growing recruitment of new HIV-infected cells as a result. The integration of HIV into the genes of the host cell explains why we cannot anticipate the development of drugs that would completely eliminate the virus from an infected individual. But this is not the major problem. Throughout our lives we harbor many other viruses, including our own endogenous retroviruses, in a silent or "latent" form without any resulting ill effects. If we could prevent the breakdown of the immune system, HIV infection might not present any serious problem.

Most current drug development programs are aimed at the prevention of viral expansion in the infected organism by decreasing the recruitment of newly infected cells, thereby postponing the development of clinical AIDS. If enough effective drugs were to become available against AIDS, infected individuals might be able to live a normal life without ever developing the disease, although life-long medication would probably be necessary.

How are effective drugs developed? At the time of the congress, there was only one definitely useful drug, AZT. It impairs the action of reverse transcriptase, the obvious first target for therapeutic attempts. Reverse transcriptase and its mechanism of action were well understood from the experience with other retroviruses, especially those that cause leukemia in mice and chickens and breast cancer in mice. Normal cells have no reverse transcriptase, and AZT is therefore able to arrest viral replication very specifically. If it were possible to shut off reverse transcriptase completely and permanently, the spread of the virus to new cells would be prevented. But a raging fire cannot be extinguished with a bucket of water. One drug alone is not sufficient to keep the virus in check for many years and even decades. High levels of AZT cannot be maintained continuously in the blood and other tissues without damage to the organs, and the drug also doesn't necessarily reach all infected cells. In spite of these serious limitations, AZT is nevertheless able to interfere with virus replication. It doesn't cure the disease, but it does prolong survival. It is now necessary to develop more powerful and more long-acting drugs against the reverse transcriptase and/or other viral products. The smaller genes of the virus also offer potential targets for therapy. Let's have a look at some of these.

HIV is a very sophisticated virus. In fact, all viruses are sophisticated. When you start to understand their strategy in some detail, you will be tenpted to say that even a relatively simple virus is more sophisticated than the most clever virologist. You will find the most advanced strategies among the viruses that can lie latent during long periods of time, and area also able to "switch on" virus production when it serves the interests of viral survival. As I have already mentioned, HIV obviously belongs to this class of viruses.

Until recently, it had been thought that the relatively small retroviruses did not have room for more that the three genes already mentioned: *gag, pol,* and *env.* If you read the complete text of the linear viral RNA code as we know it today, just as you read this text, there is no additional space, except for some regulatory "switch" regions at both ends of the molecule. But it has been shown that HIV, like a few other retroviruses of the same size, is able to express the code of its genetic text in several different manners. As a result, the single short RNA molecule carries considerably more information than meets the eye on super-ficial examination.

The virus has two different mechanisms for using certain por-tions of its genetic text twice or even more times. One is analogous to the sort of word puzzle found in all cultures that have devel-oped phonetically written languages. If you start reading the text at a certain letter and group the letters together in a certain way, you derive one set of words. Alternatively, by beginning at a different letter and by using another method of grouping the letters, a completely different word or string of words is produced.

The genetic alphabet is constructed on the basis of a three-letter code. The basic letters of both DNA and RNA are read in groups of three, and each three-letter code stands for one of the twenty-two amino acids, the building blocks of proteins, or designates a starting or stop signal. The enzymatic machinery that translates the genetic code language into the concrete protein products can therefore utilize three different reading frames, depending on where the reading begins. A sequence that can be represented as A B C D E F G H I . . . therefore produces entirely different messages when you start reading at A, B, or C, respectively, and then proceed in groups of three. If you begin with D, you are back to the same reading frame as if you had started from A.

Cells have a large surplus of DNA, much more than would be needed for all genes. A great deal of the cellular DNA is junk and doesn't code for anything.[6] Because there is no shortage of space, the cells can afford to read their genes in only one of the three possible frames. If you start reading at the letter A as in the model above, you obtain words that are linked together as a functional protein "sentence." If you start at B or C, you obtain nonsense, comparable to what a child would produce by playing with a typewriter, randomly mixing letters and punctuation marks.

Viral DNA or RNA must be used more economically than the cell's DNA, because its length is limited by what can be squeezed into the small virus particle. In some instances the virus evolution has circumvented this limitation by producing meaningful texts in two and sometimes in all three reading frames. The different messages code for different proteins. It is as if a sentence would make sense in both English and Sanskrit, by grouping the letters differently. The two texts would have different meanings, but both would make sense in the same context.

In addition to this shift in reading frame, HIV and several other viruses make more frequent use of another, more flexible mechanism to exploit their genetic text in more than one way. It is called "alternative splicing." DNA sends out instructions to the cellular protein-synthesizing factory in the form of RNA molecules called "messenger RNA." When these molecules leave the cell nucleus, they are modified by a process called "splicing." This is not the same as the phrase "gene splicing," commonly used in the media to describe genetic technology. It refers to a normal event that takes place continuously in all cells. Imagine a stretch of text written on a strip of paper. Take a pair of scissors, cut up the text, throw away certain pieces, and paste together the remaining pieces until you produce new words with new meanings. If you have been clever and have a suitable text, you can start with several copies of the original words and cut them up in different ways to produce different meanings from the same basic starting text. That is what many viruses do, and that is what HIV does.

The development of molecular biology has led us away from the concept of "one gene, one protein" that was formulated at a time when molecular genetics was still in its infancy. Now that we understand that the same RNA or DNA text can be read and/or processed in many different ways, we use the word "gene" to designate a DNA sequence that codes for a given protein. In a stricter sense, the word refers to the nucleic acid sequence that codes for a certain protein after it has been read in the correct reading frame for that particular protein and spliced in the correct way. Our modern concept of the gene thus corresponds to the final processed form of messenger RNA, or rather its DNA copy.

HIV has four known minor genes that correspond to this definition of processed genetic information. It is possible that even more such genes exist, but so far they have not been identified. Very little is known about their function in the infected organism, but laboratory studies indicate that these "minigenes" may play an important role in regulating the expression of the major viral genes. The best-known minor gene, called *tat*, can trigger the production of new virus. Like reverse transcriptase, *tat* is therefore probably a suitable target for antiviral drugs. Another minor gene has the opposite effect: it shuts down most of the viral genes.

The minor genes probably play a key role for the choice between viral latency and viral replication with the resulting production of new virus particles in a given cell. It is presumed that these genes are expressed in different ways in different cell types. One can safely assume that HIV, like other latent viruses, utilizes the normal cellular gene regulation signals to control the expression of its own genes.

As discussed in the previous chapter, cells of different types, such as lymphocytes, liver cells, muscle cells, macrophages, and nerve cells, utilize different portions of the total genetic material. They open different windows in the same house. The cells turn on a selected group of genes with the help of specialized protein molecules that bind to specific signal regions of the DNA very close to the target gene. Every regulatory protein recognizes a different sequence on the DNA. Viruses that have developed the ability to remain "invisible" in a particular cell type, unrecognized by the immune system, may utilize the same regulatory proteins to turn on or off some of their own genes. The virus did not have to learn molecular biology to know how to use the cell's regulatory proteins for its own purposes. Rather, the virus has survived in cells that happened to contain regulatory proteins that could bind to viral nucleic acid sequences, and thereby switched certain viral genes on or off. In some cases, this binding happened to help the virus to avoid the host immune response or replicate at a favorable time or place. Viral adaptation to a new type of host cell or species usually starts with a crude, approximate adaptation followed by additional mutations that enhance the ability of the virus to persist in the latent form and to spread its genome to new hosts.

I have sketched a certain scenario, but I must point out that we know very little about the regulation of HIV in cells of different types. Research concentrates on the most important known sites that can harbor HIV—the lymphocytes and macrophages and the nervous system. It is important to map the viral functions in all these cells and also in the additional, as yet unidentified cell types where the virus may persist.

Why is it so important to clarify the viral strategy in such great detail? Shouldn't we rather put all of our energy into the development of an effective vaccine that can prevent infection in the first place? Could we not then forget this horrible creature, just as we have transformed the demons of the black death and smallpox into mere paper tigers, historical fossils that occupy the dustiest shelves in the library?

No, we cannot get away so easily. HIV is too well armed against our immune response. It behaves like a minisubmarine that can invade enemy waters without being recognized. It lies on the bottom, breaks through the antisubmarine net, sends frogmen ashore, and makes a laughingstock of the invaded country and its presumably invincible navy. The virus pays no attention to the immune reactions mobilized against it outside of its safe haven. It hides in the cell nucleus, hibernates in the chromosomes, inserts itself among the cell's own genes. Here it can survive much longer than the submarine. Even the most highly advanced sub is primitive when compared with a virus like HIV.

How could one attack a miniature sub lying in the deepest waters, how can one reach a virus inside the chromosomes of a cell? You have to search for weapons that can find the ship's hull, identify its material and distinguish it from the surrounding rocks and debris. A virus integrated into the cell's DNA offers even fewer targets than a submarine. It is like a small piece of text in the memory of a word processor. The text contains the blueprint for a product to be manufactured sometime in the unspecified future. But the factory is shut down most of the time, the machinery idle, the windows covered. Isn't anything going on in this sleeping factory, any hidden activity that could become a target?

A virus that has perfected its parasitic adaptation to remain latent in cells for prolonged periods may use host cell proteins to keep its own genes shut off. This ideal situation is like the minisubmarine that has turned down its engines and disconnected its batteries. The virus can cope better than the sub, because it can supply all its need from the host cell. But its adaptation is usually not that perfect. The virus usually ensures its latency by expressing at least one of its proteins. In the best-characterized bacterial virus system, such proteins are called "repressors." They bind to the other viral genes and keep them firmly shut down to rule out the slightest possibility of their slipping into a state of uncontrolled virus production.

To attack a cell harboring a latent virus, you would have to aim at the proteins the virus produces in the latent state. A possible candidate is the HIV repressor protein that shuts off the rest of the viral genome in test-tube systems. It is not yet known whether such a protein is expressed in virus-carrying cells of the body. If that were the case, it would be an obvious target for an "immunological weapon" that could make a valuable addition to the collection of drugs that interfere with virus production.

Future therapy of HIV-infected people may come to resemble our present therapy for childhood leukemia. When I was a medical student, childhood leukemia was a disease with 100 percent mortality. The diagnosis itself was regarded as a death sentence. Now, about half of all children with leukemia are cured. This is not due to one or a few selective drugs that could interfere with essential life processes of leukemia cells without harming normal cells, as one orginally hoped. Rather, we have learned to combine several cell poisons that stop cell division by different mechanisms so that they damage the leukemic cells more than normal cells. This approach does not correspond to Paul Ehrlich's dream, a "silver bullet," or *terapia sterilisans magna*, a selective and specific sterilizing drug. A relatively unpretentious and patient collaboration between many investigators has nevertheless succeeded in curing many leukemic children and allowing them to grow up to live normal lives.

Thoughts on the Possible Future Course of the Epidemic

The most important questions concern the virulence of the HIV virus, its ability to cause disease and the possibility of inhibiting its spread within human populations. Pessimists compared the situation with that of the Titanic immediately after its collision with the iceberg, when the passengers continued dancing. Proponents of the opposite point of view argued that the panic is exaggerated, that the epidemic is about to abate, that AIDS is not really a problem of global significance. Between the lines, one could sometimes discern a conscious or subconscious distinction between "us" and "them." At its worst, it was reminiscent of the more traditional forms of discrimination based on race, ethnic identity, social status, or sexual preference. Everyone agreed that the catastrophe in Africa was a fact, but not so many cared about it, as long as it did not directly threaten the rest of the world. Despite all the expressions of sympathy for sub-Saharan Africa, and in marked contrast to the universal verbal condemnation of South Africa, there were very few voices expressing a real willingness to take meaningful action. The path to true solidarity seems still to be very long.

An Uncomfortable Subject

In the foreword to his last book, *The Drowned and the Saved* (*I soccorsi ed i salvati*), Primo Levi writes that the tendency to conceal—or when that becomes impossible, to beautify—unpleasant truths is a natural part of our civilization. The unwritten rule of silence that was obeyed by most who knew about the holocaust during the war is only an extreme example of a universal psychological phenomenon. Many aspects of sexuality; slightly (or not so slightly) unclean affairs, embarrassing and degrading both to individuals and nations; various kinds of discrimination; and indifference to the suffering of others are some of the subjects that tend to call up euphemisms rather than realistic descriptions. The early panic about the AIDS epidemic has elicited some typically fascistic responses in countries throughout the world, including Sweden and the United States. Now that AIDS has joined the spectrum of "accepted" diseases, we condemn those who try to discriminate against HIV-infected people. This is a very positive development, but the road from an essentially liberal attitude to one of true sympathy with those who have been infected by the virus or with the sick and the dying is long and arduous, especially when the victims belong to a culturally or socially alien group.

What facts can be used to build a reasonably realistic picture of the future of the epidemic from the virological and epidemiological point of view? Very few, if any. It is not possible to predict the direction in which the virus may evolve, and it is not yet clear whether the campaign of public information and education will have a serious effect on the dissemination of the virus. Viruses are subject to the same rules of mutation and natural selection as all other living organisms. The course of viral evolution can change the nature of the epidemic over time. In the worst case, the infectivity of the virus can increase, although there is no reason to expect that it will take on new modes of transmission. The opposite development is more likely. Highly pathogenic viruses generally survive less well than mutants that are not as infectious but that cause little or no disease. Viruses that have managed to infect almost all humans have often adapted themselves to an increasingly nonpathogenic relationship with their host, although this may have taken a long time. I have given examples of this elsewhere.[7] The perfectly adapted virus causes no symptoms. Viral survival is best enhanced by the appearance of increasingly infectious mutants that are less and less able to produce disease. Such a weakened virus can function as a "live vaccine" by protecting the host against the more virulent forms of the same virus that may ultimately disappear.

So much about the distant future. Right now HIV is an extremely lethal virus and it will continue to be so during the foreseeable future, at least in an untreated state. Therefore, the most important task is to stop its spread. The question is whether our many educational and informational campaigns will be effective, and in this regard there is still a great deal of uncertainty even though there are some glimmerings of light. The problem of transmission of the virus through medical procedures such as the transfusion of blood or blood products is now largely under control. Epidemiological data show that the high-risk homosexual groups in the worst-affected areas, primarily New York and San Francisco, have changed to less risky behavior. There is no clear evidence for similar changes in areas of lower AIDS incidence. A major impact is not felt until AIDS has struck people in the immediate social environment.

The spread of the disease among drug addicts seems to be an even greater problem. Some of these people are in the process of slowly committing suicide, and it is doubtful that they can care about a disease that will be fatal in the more or less distant future while they are focused on their immediate need for drugs. Many AIDS doctors believe that it is society's obligation to provide addicts with clean needles. In many areas, including Sweden and the United States, this has caused problems. Responsible authorities do not want to give mixed messages—there is conflict between the battle against drugs and attempts to prevent the spread of HIV among drug addicts. From an epidemiological point of view, it is obvious that meeting the deadly threat of the AIDS epidemic must be given the highest priority. Also, there is no evidence that the lack of clean needles can decrease or prevent drug addiction.

Another great unknown concerns the heterosexual majority. Transmission from males to females is the predominant mode of infection in Africa, whereas in industrial countries the frequency of heterosexual transmission is low. But we must understand that the virus is here to stay, and we must therefore count on a slow and cumulative rise in the number of victims among heterosexuals unless preventive measures are put into effect.can the phenomenon of heterosexual transmission be affected by information, education, or changes in our social norms? That is certainly possible to some extent. But we must realize that the effectiveness of these steps is limited, even under ideal conditions. The experience with smoking and lung cancer is somewhat relevant in this connection. Lung cancer is often a fatal and always an extremely unpleasant disease. But the causative effect of cigarette smoking has been known for more than four decades. And yet, even today, one third of human cancers, and not only lung cancer, are caused by smoking. School educational programs have decreased smoking among boys, but they have had no apparent effect on girls. Social and psychological factors seem to take priority over rational considerations.

This experience offers little support for the overly optimistic expectation that educational programs can have a major impact on heterosexual behavior. Even if the threat is presented in its true dimensions, emphasizing the more pessimistic future alternatives, education campaigns collide with the most powerful human drive. Have people not risked unwanted pregnancies since time immemorial, even in times when an unmarried woman with a child risked stigmatization and ostracization? How often have people knowingly chosen a path that has destroyed a woman's future and could lead directly to illness and death? Can you expect everybody to stay rational and consider precautions when those moments of Faulkner's "sweet cloudy fire" or the "*dolce ardor*" of the Italian renaissance take possession of one's entire being? Haven't our instincts developed to make it sure that precisely this occurs, haven't our genes and our species itself survived because of our sex drive? Isn't much of our classical literature concerned with deadly risks that lovers have been willing to take throughout time? Romeo and Juliet are much more than a remote symbol. They represent the ever-present force of nature that claims priority above all else. Paolo and Francesca may have an even greater symbolic value: they risked not only the violent death that was awaiting them, but also eternal damnation in hell, a fate they were fully expecting and that stands out so clearly in Dante's epic.

Sometimes I wonder if the education optimists are still living in a pre-Freudian era, if they have forgotten their own experiences, or if they are merely resorting to the usual double-talk of politics and the Church. It may be objected that educational programs are not addressed primarily to today's equivalents of Romeo and Juliet. A great deal could be achieved by reducing casual contacts. It would be most important and probably easiest to modify the behavior of the professional and routine practitioners of anonymous sex, prostitutes and the promiscuous. It is among these groups that the educational program could make a major impact, if the epidemic were to continue and the campaign pursued as intensively as now. There is, however, always the risk that the intensity of the program will fade through wishful thinking. We have already seen numerous waves of unjustified optimism when some "expert" announces statistical data that fail to show the expected increase in AIDS incidence (as if it were possible to predict such an expected increase), or when the answer of the "expert" is interpreted or distorted to suggest that the threat was exaggerated. It's like predicting the weather two or three years from now. This constant tendency to blare an "all clear" message reminds me of the heavy smoker grasping at every opportunity to avoid seeing reality. But unlike cigarette smoke, which injures mainly the smokers themselves, HIV enters the DNA of the species, the "holy substance of life" as exaggerated debates on biotechnology sometimes exclaim in horror—not realizing that it is precisely this technology that offers the best prospects for gaining control over HIV. There is a great danger in short-sighted optimism in the face of an everlasting virus such as HIV.

Epilogue

There is a time to be born.
There is a time to die.
Ecclesiastes 3:2

The Spring 1989 issue of the journal *Daedalus* (vol. 118, no. 2) is entitled, "Living with AIDS." This highly readable volume contains articles about AIDS, presented in historical perspective: the challenge posed by AIDS to biomedical research and health care, and the international collaborative studies in epidemiology and information exchange. But there are also a couple of articles dealing with the plight of the victims, the sick and the dying. The chapter by Paul Farmer and Arthur Kleinman entitled "AIDS as Human Suffering" contains several case reports that spotlight the highly developed medical technology of our society and its underdeveloped capacity for taking care of mortally ill patients.

Robert was a forty-four-year-old man with AIDS. He had been treated with all the advanced technology that a modern American teaching hospital at a first-class university has to offer. When his illness was already far advanced, he developed severe breathing difficulties. They were caused by a lung infection with an organism that is harmless to persons with a normal immune system but against which AIDS patients have no defense. He was treated according to a series of protocols, called algorithms. These are a series of choices among different treatment alternatives, often presented in diagrammatic form. Such algorithms help physicians make diagnoses and select programs for treatment. Robert's chest X-ray indicated that his respiratory distress was caused by the parasite Pneumocystis carinii, a common infection in AIDS patients. The infection was treated, but Robert did not improve. His fever increased and his condition worsened. Several days later he developed trismus. He previously had a fungal infection in his mouth, common in AIDS patients, that had now spread down his throat, into his pharynx and esophagus. Because he could not open his mouth, the usual protocol for esophagitis could not be followed. A specialist was consulted about the possibility of putting a tube into his stomach, but Robert refused it. He had refused a similar procedure when he was first admitted.

There are no options in the protocols for the case of patient refusal. The physicians now raised the question of whether Robert was in full command of his mental faculties. Had AIDS also infected his brain, was he suffering from AIDS dementia? One member of the medical team pointed out that Robert's case was "not included in the program," and another declared that Robert had"reached the end of the algorithm." But the others disagreed. More diagnostic tests were recommended: esophagoscopy with a biopsy and culture, a CT scan of the throat and head, repeated blood cultures, a neurological consultation. When these options were mentioned to Robert, his wordless gaze changed to an expression of anger and despair. The doctors glanced uncomfortably at each other. Their suspicions were quickly confirmed. Robert wrote on a scrap of paper: "I don't want any treatment. I just want to be kept clean."

No, is was not to be that simple. Robert got a good deal more than he asked for—the feeding tube, the endoscopy, and the CT scan. The physicians felt that they could not withhold any routine diagnostic or therapeutic intervention. Robert died within several hours of the last examination.

His physicians acted according to their instructions. They regarded his case as a "diagnostic dilemma" and a "compliance problem." Farmer and Kleinman point out that this kind of terminology illustrates a common dilemma in present-day American culture (and in the culture of other Western societies, one is tempted to add). Of course, other physicians might have acted differently.

Anitha was the daughter of a poor peasant family in Haiti. The family lived on the edge of starvation, and Anitha's childhood was filled with her parents' arguments over food. Her mother died of tuberculosis when Anitha was thirteen. Her father became an alcoholic, and Anitha fled to the city. At first she worked as a maid for a family, but soon she was out of a job and moved in with a distant relative, a sort of aunt, living in the slums. There she met

Vincent, who worked at the airport off and on, whenever help was needed. Anitha was fifteen when she accepted Vincent's suggestion that she move in with him, into a shack he set up in the same neighborhood. Anitha cooked and washed and waited for him every night. When Vincent became ill, Anitha nursed him just as she had taken care of her mother. He lost his appetite and had night sweats, swollen lymph nodes, and debilitating diarrhea. They went to doctors, witch doctors, and charlatans. They tried herbal medicines and prayers. They thought that one of the men at the airport who wanted Vincent's job had put a curse on him. They went to the voodoo priest and followed his instructions, to no avail. Vincent died. During the same time, Anitha felt very sick, and she could hardly get out of bed. Nevertheless, she set off for her home town, but she collapsed in a small village along the way. She was taken in by a woman who lived near the road. She stayed for a month, unable to walk, until her father arrived to take her home. He was a friendly man, but was severely depressed and broken down. He lived in a hut with one room, a dirt floor, and a leaky roof. It was not a place for a sick woman to live. Anitha's godmother, honoring a vow of twenty years, made room for Anitha in her overcrowded but dry house.

At first Anitha was diagnosed as having tuberculosis, and she improved with anti-tuberculosis therapy. But six months later she became ill again. A doctor confirmed that she had AIDS, but only Anita's father and godmother were informed. The godmother knew that AIDS was an infectious disease, that it could be spread with the blood of an infected person, and that it was incurable. But she was not afraid to care for Anitha, and she was adamant that Anitha not be told of her diagnosis. "It would only make her suffer more," she said. It was suggested that Anitha be taken to the AIDS clinic in the capital. The godmother refused, saying that "she will not get better there, and she will suffer from the heat and the humiliation. She won't be able to find a cool place to lie down. She will be given a pill or an injection to make her feel better for a short while. I can treat her better than that."

And that is exactly what she proceeded to do. She saw to it that Anitha sat up every day, and she made nourishing soups for her. She kept her clean and gave her the family's only sheets. She gave Anitha her own pillow and used a sack stuffed with rags for herself.

The only thing she asked from the clinic was a "nice soft wool blanket that would not irritate the child's skin."

The authors of the article interviewed the godmother, and quote her words:

"For some people, a decent death is as important as a decent life. The child has had a hard life. It is important that she be cleansed of any bitterness and regret before she dies."

Anitha herself was very calm and philosophical. Although she never mentioned AIDS by name, she did speak about "diseases from which you cannot escape." She understood that she caught the disease from Vincent, but she talked about him with love. She didn't want to be taken to a hospital. She enjoyed listening to the radio, music, and the news, and loved the woolen blanket. She was especially thankful that the authors were willing to listen to the story of her life for a few hours, before she was about to die.

The cases of Robert and Anitha say much more than the mere facts. They provide a sharp illustration of the cultural contrasts. Our Western culture had become more and more dependent on technology. One of Robert's physicians remarked ironically that, "when you're at Disney World, you take all the rides." But the problems of AIDS cannot be solved by technology at present. The demands are at a different level, one that our culture is not prepared to meet. We rarely ask the question how our illusory world relates to the realities of disease and death.

For Farmer and Kleinman, it is especially ironic that everyone seemed to be so concerned with Robert's personal rights in the impersonal environment of the American hospital. They see it as a detached and cool bioethical attention to abstract individual rights rather than an affirmation of humane responses to specific existential needs. It is especially ironic that Robert's "lonely death, so rich in all the technology applied to his last hours, could be so poor in all those supportive human virtues that resonate from the poverty-stricken village where Anitha died among friends."

One reason for our relative inability to deal with the deadly reality of AIDS lies in the hypocritical attitude of our culture toward death, reflected by the general tendency to use euphemisms to describe our mortality. The constant preoccupation with machines, the tests and further therapeutic planning in situations where there is no therapy, reveals that we see death as the greatest evil and is a part of the general euphemistic denial of our mortality. It is a continuous, hopeless attempt to escape the only certain conclusion that we can draw. We have obviously lost touch with our most important reality. Nevertheless, the devoted and committed voluntary support groups that take care of AIDS patients in San Francisco and other places demonstrate that at least a small number of people, often among the patients' closest friends, are both willing and able to establish contact with this reality and then do extraordinary work.

I have previously written about the Swiss law professor Peter Noll. [8] Although he had an approximately 30 percent chance of being cured of his bladder cancer, he resolutely declined all treatment. He did not feel that the quality of his life after a radical operation would be consistent with his attitudes about life and death.[9] He preferred to spend his time as a free human being, not as a prisoner of hospital routines and treatments. He wanted to use his limited remaining time to remind us, with Montaigne and Seneca as his models, that only the awareness of death can give our lives the meaning, joy, and dignity that we are striving for. He devoted his nine remaining months to the encounter with his death and the process of his dying. His last months included "a great deal of sorrow, but also real bliss and, surprisingly enough, no despair whatsoever."

Noll reexamined his resolve continously while he was writing the book that he left us. He was not seeking consultation and did not want to extend his life within the remembrance of others, a usual but meaningless effort to linger on a bit longer. Rather, he wanted to describe his experiences in a situation that can befall any one of us at any time. Most of all, he wanted to convey a most important insight—that it is most sensible to deal with the problems of death and dying while one is still in the best health. He went so far as to praise the dreaded death from cancer, since it offers enough time to contemplate and to become intimately acquainted with death. Noll stressed that we would live a better and more civilized life if we were to live it as it is, with a constant awareness of our limited time. Its exact duration is of no importance, since none of us can achieve immortality. We are all in the same boat. The only difference is that Noll knew approximately when he was to leave this world, while the rest of us live on in blessed or troubled uncertainty.

Just as Peter Noll was reminded of his mortality when he learned that he had cancer, the AIDS epidemic has reminded us of our vulnerability, the precariousness of our situation, and the transience of our individual present. It moves to the forefront a truth that our species has known throughout its history, but that we have done our very best to forget—that suffering is a central and ever-present part of our existence.

Part Six

9

Pietà

....*Aber einmal sah*
er noch des Mädchens Antlitz, das sich wandte
mit einem Lächeln, hell wie eine Hoffnung,
die beinah ein Versprechen war: erwachsen
zurückzukommen aus dem tiefen Tode
zu ihm dem Lebenden - Da schlug er jäh
die Hände vors Gesicht, wie er so kniete,
um nichts zu sehen mehr nach diesem Lächeln.

But yet once more he saw the maiden's
face, that turned to him, smiling a smile as
radiant as a hope, that was almost a
promise: to return, grown up, out of the
depths of death again, to him, the living—
Thereupon he flung his hands, as he
knelt there, before his face, so as to see no
more after that smile.

Rainer Maria Rilke, *Alcestis* [1]

As I walk through the Christian quarter of Jerusalem, I catch sight
of an inscription just under a relief of the crucified Christ over
the entrance to a monastery. I read it absentmindedly, more or
less to test my rusty high school Latin. I find to my surprise that
I am moved by the words. I stand there reading for a short while,
and soon I know the words by heart: *O vos omnes, qui transitis per*
viam, attendite et videte si est dolor sicut dolor meus. [2] (All you who pass
this way, look and see: is there any sorrow like the sorrow that
afflicts me.) The origin of the Latin text could easily be traced
to a direct translation of the original Hebrew text of the prophet
Jeremiah's lamentations over Jerusalem-Zion, while captive in
Babylonia.

Why am I so deeply affected by these words? I don't believe in the crucified, in any God or his son, no matter what language they use when they try to speak to me. And yet . . .[2]
Misericordia. Compassion with the dying. The anguish of being carried too far, repudiation, denial, and flight. *Pietà,* the unattainable—forever attracting, always betrayed. Ionesco has said that only our loneliness in the face of death unites all of us. Unites us, yes; abandons us, yes. *Miserere nobis . . .*

How deeply can we immerse ourselves in the pain of the dying without succumbing with them?

Rilke's deepest compassion is addressed to his God, but who is his God, the constantly recurring "You" of his "Stundenbuch"[3]— who is his God if not man himself?

Du bist der Arme, du der Mittellose,
du bist der Stein, der keine Stätte hat,
du bist der fortgeworfene Leprose,
der mit der Klapper umgeht vor der Stadt.

You're the poor man, the utterly denuded,
you are the stone for which no place was found,
you are the leper whom the town excluded,
before the gates he rattles on his round.

Denn dein ist nichts, so wenig wie des Windes
und deine Blösse kaum bedekt der Ruhm;
das Alltagskleidchen eines Waisenkindes
ist herrlicher und wie ein Eigentum.

For, like the wind, you're wholly unpossessive,
and all your fame scarce hides your nakedness;
an orphan's week-day wear is more impressive
and something he seems really to possess.

Du bist so arm wie eines Keimes Kraft
in einem Mädchen, das es gern verbürge
und sich die Lenden presst, dass sie erwürge
das erste Atmen ihrer Schwangerschaft.

You're poor as the seed's strength but recently
sprung in a girl who'd not be seen a mother
and, pressing in her thighs, attempts to smother
the earliest breathing of her pregnancy.

Und du bist arm: so wie der Frühlingsregen,
der selig auf der Städte Dächer fällt,
und wie ein Wunsch, wenn Sträflinge ihn hegen
in einer Zelle, ewig ohne Welt.
Und wie die Kranken, die sich anders legen

und glücklich sind, wie Blumen in Geleisen
so traurig arm im irren Wind der Reisen,
und wie die Hand, in die man weint, so arm.

And you're as poor as is the vernal rain
that falls on city roofs so blissfully,
and as some wish that prisoners retain
within their cells, unrealisably.
And as the sick, who, turning yet again,
are happy; as the flowers in railroad gravel,
so sadly poor in passing gusts of travel;
and poor as is the hand we weep into . . .

Und was sind Vögel gegen dich, die frieren,
was ist ein Hund, der tagelang nicht frass,
und was ist gegen dich das Sichverlieren,
das stille, lange Traurigsein von Tieren,
die man als Eingefangene vergass?

And how can even freezing birds compare
with you, or dogs unfed the livelong day,
and what, compared with you, is the despair
of sad dumb creatures fastened in somewhere
by some forgetter who has gone away?

Und alle Armen in den Nachtasylen,
was sind sie gegen dich und deine Not?
Sie sind nur kleine Steine, keine Mühlen,
aber sie mahlen doch ein ewig Brot.

And what are all the paupers, nightly filling
the shelters, when we think what you survive?
They're only little stones, not mills, though milling
a little bread to keep themselves alive.

Du aber bist der tiefste Mittellose,
der Bettler mit verborgenem Gesicht;
du bist der Armut grosse Rose,
die ewige Metamorphose
des Goldes in das Sonnenlicht.

You've reached a deeper depth of desolation,
the beggar with the hidden countenance;
you're poverty's great consummation,
the everlasting transmutation
of gold into the sun's own radiance.

Du bist der leise Heimatlose,
der nicht mehr einging in die Welt;
zu gross und schwer zu jeglichem Bedarfe.
Du heulst im Sturm. Du bist wie eine Harfe,
an welcher jeder Spielende zerschällt.

Beyond this world's accommodation,
in silent homelessness you stand:
too great and hard for all that men require.
You howl in storms. You're like a lyre
on which is shattered every playing hand.

Who are you, you rejected leper, that magnificent rose of the destitute, the hand into which we weep; you whose glory barely covers your shame, you who own little more than the wind, you the harp that destroys all who play upon you? Are you my own suffering, or are you my anguish at not being able to feel the suffering of others?

Hiroshima 1987, Peace Square

A sudden idea, an unplanned stop. Earlier in the day in my hotel room in Okayama, I had gone over my itinerary. Fukuoka was the next scheduled stop on my lecture tour. But my finger, moving casually along the railway route on the map, came to a sudden halt, as if at a stop sign. A signal emanated from the map that shocked my entire system. No, I hadn't misread, it wasn't a mistake that might be corrected with stronger eyeglasses. There it was, HIROSHIMA, amid the other genteel names—Kyoto with its cherry blossoms, Nikko with its golden temples, Nara with its many ancient statues of Buddha. But suddenly none of these names could help any longer. Even Tokyo faded quickly—its pliant, earthquake-resistant skyscrapers, its thousands of identical shops with the latest cameras and ever more sophisticated Walkmans; they all vanished as if they had never existed. I sought in vain to take refuge in my memories of Hamamatsu and the unbelievable Yamaha factory that I had just visited. Can you imagine that they spit out seventy big concert grand pianos every day, and they run music schools with 170,000 students, all over Japan! No sense even trying. The entire attractive, frightening miracle of present-day Japan, this unique hybrid of the antique and the modern, fell away suddenly as if through a trap door. Only a single word remained: Hiroshima.

What female voice utters the Japanese name with a French accent; who is the man who responds in French with a Japanese accent? Why do I see the two naked bodies sliding over, around, and under each other—large, glistening, moist expanses of skin? What voices do I hear, talking to each other, passing by each other without meeting, in the hot tub, in the wide, white bed during an endlessly long but accidentally temporary night of love? *"Tu n'as rien vu à Hiroshima,"* he says with his strange accent, says it over and over again while they embrace. His voice answers first, answers and meets it, passes by, enters, avoids, meets, and fails to meet her nightmare, a vision whispered in perfect French, whispered and repeated, meets and is met, does not meet, passes by.[4]

"Tu n'as rien vu à Hiroshima. Rien."
You saw nothing in Hiroshima. Nothing.
I have seen everything. Everything. The burned iron, the shattered iron, iron made as vulnerable as flesh. Stones, burned stones, shattered stones.
Ten thousand degrees at Peace Square.
The temperature of the sun at Peace Square.
You saw nothing in Hiroshima.
Two hundred thousand dead.
Eighty thousand injured.
In nine seconds.
You saw nothing. Nothing.

We are standing in front of a window in the tidy museum, looking at the iron that became as vulnerable as flesh, at the stone that shattered as if made of porcelain.

Do we really see it? No, we see nothing. We saw nothing in Hiroshima.

Large buses are coming and going. Groups of schoolchildren from all over Japan visit Hiroshima every day—girls and boys, between fifteen and seventeen, dressed in crisp, proper uniforms. They radiate the Japanese combination of discipline and intensity—apart from that, they could be students from anywhere. They talk, laugh, and eat ice cream as soon as they come out of the building. But one girl suddenly covers her eyes with her hands—she doesn't want to see more. Another turns away and begins to cry.

We are drinking coffee with our Japanese colleague from Okayama who wanted to accompany us. He had been the first Japanese to join us as a visiting scientist in the Tumor Biology Laboratory twenty-five years earlier. We have often talked about many things other than science, but never about the war and certainly never about Hiroshima. I find it difficult to say anything. Suddenly he says, in a calm and matter-of-fact voice, as if he were discussing a trivial laboratory experiment, that he had walked seven miles through the center of the demolished city two weeks after the atomic explosion. He was looking for his brother-in-law, whom he found safe on the outskirts of the city. Because he received an unknown dose of radiation during his search, he would be qualified to register officially as a "Hiroshima survivor," but he never bothered to do so.

I still find it difficult to say anything. But again I hear his calm and almost monotonous voice: "It was absolutely necessary to drop an atomic bomb on Japan. But one bomb would have been enough."

I had never heard that from any Japanese.

"Why do you say that?"

"Most Japanese wanted to keep fighting. They had no intention of giving up the war. It could have gone on many more years, and many more would have died."

I have seen nothing in Hiroshima. But suddenly I begin to wonder if my Japanese friend has seen anything either, despite his seven-mile walk through that burned-out hell. He is probably correct, at least from an objective point of view. But how can you combine such objectivity with an attempt to fathom what none of us has experienced—the burning inferno, or even the gradual, insidious but equally terrifying death from radiation sickness?

It cannot be done. You can concentrate on only one aspect or the other. It is like looking at Escher's pictures of black and white birds. You can see either the black or the white birds, but not both at the same time.

As I walked through the beautiful Peace Park, at a site directly under the hypocenter of the explosion, I was reminded of the first autopsy I attended while still a high school student, interested in the natural sciences. I watched as a human brain was lifted out of the skull and placed in front of me, in all its bareness. I was painfully aware that it was a brain that had thought and felt, just like my own. But now they were about to cut it apart as if it were no more than a bit of jelly. It was treated with no more respect than a stool sample. I stared, shocked, at the pathologist and the medical students, and at the orderly who was making crude jokes. Where had I ended up, what kind of people were these?

Some years later I had become a medical student myself, an assistant in pathology with a passionate interest in autopsies. Every corpse was a detective story for me. I tried to reconstruct the concrete facts, to identify some of the many possibilitites of life and disease that had become realities in a particular person or "case," as they were called. It was an encounter with disease, not with individual human beings. The tissue was merely material, it evoked no associations with thoughts, feelings, or suffering. It was equally impossible to identify with it as with—yes, a stool sample.

Only occasionally did those protective walls shake for a moment. I was standing in front of a female corpse with red fingernails and toenails—so unusual for those days—a body that belonged to an actress whom I had often admired, applauded, and dreamed about. I can still feel my sudden sense of shock, bordering on dizziness—she had tertiary syphilis and probably had not been in full possession of her senses for years. Despite that, her toenails were freshly polished. I can also remember the body of a great poet, an incomparable master of language, of feelings, colors, and moods, who had the cirrhotic liver of a chronic alcoholic. I thought of the scene from Hamlet with the gravediggers. A mind-reading colleague might have considered this a most inappropriate thought for a pathologist. Hamlet is holding the skull of Yorick and thinking of the times he played with him as a child.

"Where be your gibes now? your gambols? your flashes of merriment, that were wont to set the table on a roar? Not one now, to mock your own grinning? quite chapfallen? Now get you to my lady's chamber, and tell her, let her paint an inch thick, to this favour she must come."

But a moment later it was gone. The logic of the case unfolded mercilessly, sweeping over my emotions like a tidal wave that covers plants, mussels, cliffs, and islets as if they never existed. But they are there, lurking in the depths, waiting for the next low tide.

Only once did a forbidden, unprofessional, weak, shameful identification with the body on the table push aside the pathologist; it was the case of a twelve-year-old child who had died of tuberculous meningitis. I managed to finish the autopsy with my veneer intact, but thereafter I tried to avoid autopsies on children.

A couple of decades later, I learned how anatomy is taught in Iceland. Each class consists of 140 students, a tenth of whom are foreigners who do not plan to practice medicine in Iceland, and only one third of whom eventually finish their medical studies. Nevertheless, each year the whole anatomy class is sent at government expense to Liverpool, England, to spend a month doing anatomical dissections. The official reason is the lack of a sufficient number of corpses on Iceland, but it is common knowledge that there is another reason. Most Icelanders know each other or members of each other's families. It is apparently not possible to learn anatomy, to focus on the structures that are common to all members of our species—and are even further removed from the individuality of a person than is a case history—by using the body of someone you have known.

No, you cannot do it. But why not? To avoid recognizing yourself, your own inevitable future, in the corpse? Or is it to avoid compassion with his life and death, which might threaten your own defenses?

Is it possible to break through these psychological barriers? Who overcomes them, when and why? At one extreme we see the total lack of compassion, as in the Japanese writer Yukio Mishima— a glorifier of blood, strength, and death, a champion and an ultimate victim of the samurai culture, who sacrificed himself and his closest friends on its altar. To a modern observer it was a senseless act, but according to contemporary Japanese commentators, it was a logical and aesthetic fulfillment of a culture that reigned over Japanese souls for so long in the past and that still influences them heavily. At the other end of the spectrum we find the medieval monks and nuns, the ascetics and flagellants. What did they wish to beat inside themselves, what drove them to nurse the much-feared lepers, what did they wish to prove when they drank pus from abscesses? What drives Mother Theresa and all the volunteers who devote their lives to dying AIDS patients?

....*attendite et videte si est dolor sicut dolor meus.* Why do you speak to us as we pass you on our way (*transitis per viam*), whatever you happen to be called, whether it be the prophet Jeremiah, Zion the captive, or you the crucified latecomer? Why do you boast of your sorrow? Do you dare to risk the comparison that you are provoking? Will you remain above that gate after that? And will we be able to continue our journey?

Stockholm, 1962

A frail, white-haired old lady is visiting me with her son. She is a famous artist, and her name was legendary when I was growing up in Hungary. She has educated and inspired many generations of artists. Her graceful, refined movements remind me of old ladies from my childhood. Now she can barely speak because she has tongue cancer, one of the most painful of all diseases. Her physical pain, incomprehensible to an observer, raises a wall between us. I can only try to imagine the truth behind her sad but still warm smile. Her son has persuaded her to come to Stockholm in the vain hope of finding a more effective treatment.

What can I tell her? That I cannot offer anything except a routine referral to my clinical colleagues? Should I call an oncologist or a neurosurgeon who might consider severing a nerve to relieve the pain temporarily? Should I indulge in a white lie and suggest that she submit to further tests and to palliative treatment that would only prolong her suffering? Without much conviction I try, compelled by a somewhat misplaced sense of duty—or perhaps only to prove to myself that I can resist the impulse to run away, that I can defy my own fear of becoming "the hand in which you weep" (*wie die Hand, in die man weint, so arm* . . .). I explain, make some telephone calls to establish a few contacts, and try to sound as optimistic as possible. Then I look at my watch and mutter in an embarrassed tone that unfortunately I must go to a meeting. It happens to be the truth, but I still feel that it is a false excuse. She thanks me as if I had saved her life, and presents me with a small red tablecloth that she had sewn herself. I have it on my table to this day. I am looking at it as I write this. I look at it, and I see it but I don't see it; I look but I try to turn away. I am afraid to look at it too often, too long, or too intently. There, underneath the tablecloth, within the tabletop, hides her smile. It was the last I saw of her as she was leaving my room, turning her head toward me. It reflected great hope and final resignation at the same time, without contradiction. Deep within me sits The Other, wishing to throw my hands over my eyes so that I can see nothing after her smile.

....attendite et videte si est dolor sicut dolor meus.

What pain shall I compare with your suffering? I remember an article by Per Uddén in the Swedish newspaper *Dagens Nyheter* on February 8, 1966, entitled "The Child, the Doctor, and Death." "A five-year-old girl, her abdomen swollen after an unsuccessful appendectomy, asks, between vomiting attacks, 'Daddy, may I please die soon?' 'Yes, my little girl, you may.'"

Is that enough, or do you want to hear more about old ladies?

Budapest, Mid-May 1944

I am a combined errand boy and assistant secretary on the third floor of the building belonging to the Jewish Council, formerly the Jewish Community, in the center of what will soon become the Budapest ghetto, the last ghetto in Europe. My job is to keep order in the long lines of agitated people crowding outside the "housing office." The "ghettoization" has recently begun. Two to three families are forced to crowd together in every room because large parts of the city must be made "free of Jews" (*Judenfrei*) in only a few days. The people are upset, they all want to be excepted, they are seeking ways out—or at least a respite. In another line, other even more agitated people are waiting for documentation from the Jewish Council that they perform "useful work"; they are looking for pieces of paper to protect them from gunfire. I see them but I don't. None of them knows what I know. In the strictest confidence, I have just been allowed to read a report written by two young Slovakian Jews who managed to escape from Auschwitz. I know what lurks beyond the lines and the ghetto. All this is merely a smokescreen and a farce. Auschwitz-Birkenau, the largest death factory in the history of mankind, is awaiting us all— we have been condemned to death by the nation that rules over us. The crematoria are blazing day and night, the machinery is working at maximum efficiency so that we can all be "dealt with" before it is too late. Adolf Eichmann and his staff are sitting at the Hotel Astoria, only a few hundred yards from the Jewish Council.

An elderly woman comes up to me and asks, quietly and politely, if the Jewish religious community is still functioning in the building. Yes, of course it is, but it is difficult to find the office behind the masses of agitated people. What does the lady want? Well, she would like to pay the maintenance fee for the upkeep of her husband's grave. The times are difficult, and as it's not clear what is going to happen, she wants to pay for a year in advance.

I take her to the office of the religious community. She thanks me with a smile and says some startling and unforgettable words. "It feels good to have spoken with a European in this building."I think about the report of the two Slovaks. Who is a European? Where is Europe?

I know that my beloved grandmother and my uncles have already been transformed into the thick black smoke belching incessantly from the crematorium chimneys. I have a feeling that my only chance to avoid following them is both to know and not to know this fact.

It was only quite recently, as I watched Claude Lanzmann's monumental film "Shoah," that I understood the significance of this double thinking. One of the subjects being interviewed and secretly filmed by Lanzmann was an SS man from Treblinka. He was describing the "tube" (*Schlauch*) in which the naked victims were forced to wait in below-zero temperatures while those ahead were gassed to death. Without any noticeable emotion, he described how those waiting burst into tears when they heard the roaring motors that generated the slow-killing diesel fumes and the screams of the victims who preceded them, and how the fear of their imminent death overcame them. They lost control of their bowels and bladders and shivered with cold, there in the tube. Suddenly I was seized by a feeling that I had never experienced before. I realized for the first time, in precise physical detail, that this is more or less the way in which my grandmother, my uncles, and my small cousin had perished. I also understood that I am only slightly better prepared to understand how they must have felt than is the average teenager of today.

Bruno Bettelheim has written that it is impossible for anyone who has been in Auschwitz ever to be free of it. I'm not sure of that—I know several survivors who function normally. But the fate of the poet Paul Celan and the chemist and author Primo Levi is consistent with Bettelheim's suggestion that the "shadow of Auschwitz" finally caught up with them when they committed suicide. But who knows that this is true? Our defenses against approaching the unbearable too closely probably have a great survival value. But we cannot retain our humanity unless we try to mount a defense against this defense.

Gångsätra Public Bath, Lidingö, Sweden, 1980

It is time for my daily monotonous swimming routine. I go into the sauna with full battle gear: reliable earplugs, strong eyeglasses, and under my arm, a large brown envelope containing my endless paperwork. I am looking forward to a few minutes of uninterrupted concentration. The light is very dim, as many of my sauna colleagues have told me, but it's quite sufficient for my purpose. The habitués know me well, and they are no longer surprised at my peculiar habits. They have long since given up trying to penetrate my earplugs with their usual conversation about the temperature of the water, the weather, ongoing or planned construction projects, or questions about cancer research.

Barely have I plunged into the alternatingly interesting and boring world of half-finished scientific papers when one of the other guests lets out such a loud and hearty "Hi!" that my earplugs surrender.

I almost never recognize my sauna colleagues when I meet them, fully dressed, on the street. It is difficult to imagine that they have names, professions, and homes. And now it is equally difficult to recognize the naked figure standing before me, whom I had only seen fully dressed. It takes me several moments to realize that he is one of my former students, who received his degree more than ten years earlier. He has become a clinical cancer specialist. I have not seen him since he left our laboratory. In a sauna, where all is revealed, direct questions are allowed.

"Are you a good cancer doctor?"

"I certainly hope that I am now, but I wasn't when I started."

"Why not?"

"I did not know the reasons at the time, but I felt that I wasn't good. Then I took a course with Loma Feigenberg, the psychiatrist at our cancer hospital, and I realized then that I was unable to cope with my own fear of death when I was confronted with patients who were dying or doomed to die. I ran away from them, I swept them under the rug. After I came to understand that connection, I was better able to confront my own fear of death and could therefore deal with dying patients. Since that time, I have been a better doctor."

I believe him, but I wonder if it is only a question of death anxiety. The discomfort I felt at my first autopsies could have had something to do with that fear, with the constant reminder that someday I too would be lying there. But that feeling was quickly replaced by my growing professional objectivity as I became accustomed to seeing corpses and internal organs as objects of study, without constant identification with my subjective reality. After that, it wasn't nearly as difficult or painful to imagine G. K., the candidate for death, after he had managed to live successfully through all that was in store and ended up on the autopsy table. Contact with a living but fatally ill patient is completely different. It is more difficult to keep a distance when you have a living person in front of you. Empathy is a natural and desirable reaction, but it can also be seen as an imminent threat. How far does one dare go? What is the limit to true sympathy, how far can compassion reach, how much suffering can you share? At what point do polite words become empty; when do we pull the curtain to hide a lack of interest, and mount the shield that we use to protect ourselves from the real or imagined dangers of more profound involvement? How long can we endure suffering with others without succumbing ourselves?

Bombay, 1964

It is five o'clock in the morning and I am on my way to the city, on my first visit to India. As the bus reaches the outskirts of the city, I see hundreds of people sleeping on the sidewalk, with pieces of newspaper covering their faces. For some it is time to wake up. They squat for a short while, get up, shake out their rags a bit, throw away their newspapers, and go off.

As we arrive at the hotel, my car is surrounded by begging children, and I also see some emaciated old men and women stretching out their hands.

Later in the day I have lunch with an English colleague at the Naval Officers Club, in the best English colonial style. He has been working here for several years, spending five or six months at a time. I try to tell him how disturbed I am by what I had seen earlier that morning. He looks at me, surprised. When he finally understands what I am talking about, he reacts with a sort of weary "Well, one gets used to it. After a while, one doesn't notice it any longer."

Stockholm, Christmas Day, 1987

News on the radio: One million people have attended the funeral of the famous actor and politician Ramashandran in Bombay, India. Five people at the funeral committed suicide by setting themselves on fire. The police prevented several others from following their example.

Death of a Physician

Gabriel Izak, my childhood friend, a professor of hematology in Jerusalem, was known as a good physician and a strong personality.

I met him for the first time when I was nineteen, shortly after I had successfully escaped from the Nazi death trains rolling incessantly toward Auschwitz. I had no identification papers. He worked in a factory that made shoes for the German and Hungarian armies, now in retreat from the advancing Russians. He had a large collection of false identity papers and handed them out generously to friends in danger. Every night new refugees appeared at his lab. After an hour or two they had received their new identities and had to manage on their own.

Izak was not a man of many words. He could appear quite introverted and withdrawn at times, but he could nevertheless easily make contact with virtually anybody. He acted quickly, in a no-nonsense manner. That's the way things were—there was no time for tears, not even for parents, brothers, or sisters on the way to the gas chambers, perhaps already dead. We had to act quickly. We had to mobilize our unyielding will to live against the German death factories.

Only once did I see Izak upset in those days. One of his closest associates had been taken prisoner by the Arrow Cross. He was Izak's contact man with a resistance group that was completely unknown to us but which supported the operation. It wasn't until after the war that it was identified as the Labor Zionist youth movement Hashomer Hatzair. There was no doubt that our friend was going to be tortured for information on the organization and our hiding place. With lightning speed and without hesitation, Izak evacuated all thirty people living in his apartment and moved them to other locations. It proved to be unnecessary. Izak's friend had escaped by jumping from one of the tall bridges into the pitch-black, icy Danube forty feet below. He wasn't wounded by the bullets fired at him in the dark river, but his body was covered with the wounds from his previous "treatment." He swam to shore and was safe, although he contracted pneumonia. He had not betrayed us.

Both Izak and I studied medicine after the war. Our paths separated in 1947. I came to Sweden, and he went to Jerusalem. After a distinguished scientific and clinical career, he became the first professor of hematology in Israel. He was feared by some, but his staff, students, and many of his colleagues had great respect for him. The patients loved him.

Shortly after the Six Day War, I learned that he had served as chief physician of a large Hadassah hospital in Jerusalem during the war and in the weeks that followed. It was probably the most difficult position for a doctor at the time. Little or no civilian casualties were expected in Jerusalem. The war with the Egyptians was raging in the Sinai, and plans were being made for battle with the Syrians in the north. It was expected that King Hussein, caught in the middle, would remain neutral, but Jordan joined the attack by opening fire on West Jerusalem. The final three days of the war were the bloodiest that the city had experienced since the war of liberation in 1948. The Hadassah hospital was filled to capacity, with surgeons operating in the corridors. The shortage of doctors was catastrophic, as all the young doctors were at the front. Izak worked practically nonstop and had not left the hospital for two weeks. Those close to him said later that it was the first time in his life that he was seriously depressed. He couldn't bear the thought of how much needed to be done for the patients that could not be done.

Several months later, the director general of the Hadassah hospital, professor Koloman Mann, visited me in Stockholm. I mentioned that Izak was a childhood friend of mine, and I wondered if it was true that he had been chief physician during the war.

"Yes," said Mann, "I'm the one who appointed him."

"Did you choose him because you were aware of his achievements during the Second World War?"

What achievements? Mann had heard nothing about any achievements. Izak preferred to act rather than talk about his actions.

At the beginning of the 1970s, however, he suddenly wanted to tell me something, in the greatest secrecy. He began with a very unusual confession. He was carrying a great burden that he wasn't permitted to reveal. Nonetheless, he felt that he had to discuss it with a friend and colleague whom he could trust. It had to do with one of his patients, an "old woman." He used the Hungarian word *öregasszony* —we always spoke to each other in our mother tongue. This word has a certain nuance that is lost in translation. It is not quite "old lady" or "old woman," but perhaps more like "old granny." It is an everyday word, not particularly respectful but, depending on the way it is used, its overtones may remind you of fairy tales, and particularly of the archetypal old woman who turns out to have supernatural powers. The connotations depend largely on the listener's frame of mind.

This old and somehow very special woman had a lymphoma, a tumor that arises from one type of white blood cells. It was a very malignant tumor and called for aggressive therapy. Izak was used to making decisions for his patients. He never hesitated to use this authority when he knew that he was acting in their best interests. He did not have much patience with long discussions or irrational objections. But in this case the situation was different. He knew precisely what kind of treatment he wanted to give, but he had strict orders to keep the drugs at a level that would not disturb the patient's work. I was amazed. Who could give such an order? How could Izak, for the first time, allow outside demands to override his professional judgment?

The order came from the highest authority, Izak answered hesitatingly, as if he still hadn't decided whether or not he should tell me. It came from the patient herself. The "old woman" was the prime minister of Israel.

Golda Meir's illness remained a well-kept political secret. Whenever she arrived at Hadassah hospital for treatment, she was more heavily camouflaged than she was when David Ben-Gurion asked her to visit King Abdullah of Jordan in 1947, and she disguised herself as an Arab woman. The secret was kept during her entire term of office and was only revealed long after she chose to resign her post as prime minister. But before she resigned, while under stressful chemotherapy, she led Israel during the difficult October war in 1973. It is known that she made all the crucial decisions herself. Our colleague, the biochemist Efraim Katzir, who served as Israel's president during the October war, described the situation a year later, still not knowing of Golda Meir's illness:

"Among all of Israel's prime ministers, including Ben-Gurion, I have the greatest respect for Golda Meir. She knows as much about weapons, military strategy, and warfare as an ordinary housewife. Nevertheless, she is the one who directed the war. It was her decisions that averted the impending and potentially catastrophic collapse on the northern front. The generals were in a panic. The legendary defense minister had a nervous breakdown. Golda Meir listened to all of the information, reflected on it calmly and logically and then made the correct decisions."

Later, after she had stepped down from office, I met her a couple of times at Izak's home. I was completely spellbound by the "old woman," as Izak still called her in Hungarian—with her plain but articulate use of words, her wrinkled face, and the sharply focused eyes that did not stray for an instant from her conversation partner. I knew that Olof Palme had spoken of her as a "apparition from the Old Testament." Maybe so—she certainly saw the world in terms of black and white, and she didn't hesitate to make decisions accordingly. In some ways she was the mother, or the grandmother, of all Israelis. She could burst into tears when she heard about the death of someone's son in combat, whether she knew the family or not. But a moment later, she could make a decision that would bring about the death of hundreds of sons, if she thought it necessary to avert something even worse.

Izak didn't care very much for Golda Meir's politics. He considered her too rigid and doctrinaire. But during the growing doctor-patient relationship, his attitude changed gradually from skepticism to increasing sympathy, and finally to an absolute devotion to her. For the first time in his career, Izak became docile and compliant. He provided what he considered an inferior form of treatment that had no noticeable effects to the outside world and was compatible with the hard-working day of the prime minister. In spite of her widely disseminated tumor, Golda Meir had not only led the October war effort but also managed to weather the harsh storms of Israeli politics.

Strangely enough, her tumor remained more stationary than expected, not only while she was in power but also for several years afterward, while she was constantly being consulted by her successors. After that, the final collapse came quite suddenly. In the fall of 1978, Izak came to my temporary office at the immunology department in Jerusalem, looking very sad. He had just said goodbye to the "old woman." He was about to leave for a conference in Mexico, and he knew that he would never see her again. He then said something very strange, something that I had never heard him say before in any situation, not even during the worst of the Nazi times:

"Strictly speaking, I ought to stay here, but I know that I wouldn't be able to deal with it."

I remember that Izak once told me that every true doctor dies along with each dying patient. In this case, he didn't dare confront this death.

A few days later I met professor Rachmilevitz, the nestor of the Hadassah doctors and Izak's own mentor. He was one of the old and by now legendary Russian immigrant generation, a member of the close circle around Ben-Gurion and Golda Meir. He himself was suffering from an advanced cancer, but continued to attend every important lecture.

"How is Golda?"

"She is dying," he said. "I've never seen anyone die like that. It's truly remarkable—she dies just as she lived. She is in terrible pain, but she doesn't complain. She only says, 'I have lived a good life. Now it's time to suffer and to die,' and then she turns toward the wall."

Two days later, all regularly scheduled radio programs gave way to classical music. Soon thereafter came the announcement, "Golda Meir is dead."

She was buried a few days later, in pouring rain, in the presence of an enormous crowd. Friends and political foes from all levels of the thousand-faceted Israeli society stood speechless under their umbrellas. All the men wore hats in accordance with Jewish custom. There they stood, not far from the grave of the visionary Theodor Herzl and other founding fathers of the state. They stood motionless as the rain poured down.

Izak returned home a week later. His own time was also limited and he knew it. He brushed off with a laugh any questions of what he would do after retiring ten years later, saying, "That's not going to happen." After his brother, the chief surgeon in Jaffa who was ten years older than Izak, died of a heart attack in January 1980, Izak was not quite himself, but he kept his composure toward the outside world, as before. But he could no longer lift himself out from under the shadow that had fallen over him. He survived his brother by only six weeks, but managed to organize a symposium in his memory in the interim.

One day in March, he went to work as usual. He attended grand rounds but complained afterward of a feeling of fatigue. He asked to lie down and rest for a few minutes in his office. His assistants waited outside. When he didn't come out again, they looked in and found him lying on his sofa, dead of a heart attack. Like Golda, he died as he had lived.

Jerusalem, 1987

Once again I stand in front of you, reading your exhortation to us there over the monastery gate, freely and arrogantly Latinized from Jeremiah: *Attendite et videte si est dolor sicut dolor meus.* Aren't you ashamed of the translation into a later and foreign language, not your language at all? You should at least use the original words: *Habbitu ureu im jesh machov kemachovi..*

Why should I look at your suffering, whoever you are or pretend to be? Can we cope better with our own suffering if we live with your story? Can we reconcile ourselves more easily with the absurd paradoxes of our lives? Can we feel more compassion for each other if we contemplate your suffering rather than the suffering of millions, or billions, of others that we could choose instead? Can we approach our common destiny, our highly individual death, more easily? Can the contemplation of your suffering decrease violence? Yes, perhaps to some extent under the right conditions, either in particularly fortunate or "democratic" societies and sometimes even under the opposite conditions, within minority groups that live under oppressive governments. But your suffering has also been exploited for the opposite purposes. Huge, powerful states have been established and bloody wars fought in your name. The descendents of those labeled as your persecutors have been imprisoned in ghettos, deported, and gassed not sevenfold, not seven times sevenfold, but a millionfold. Do you dare look on us and on our suffering? Was it so easy to dissociate compassion, your allegedly new, seemingly triumphant notion, from its practical implementation—could it not prevent humans from turning against other humans like wolves, exactly as before? How is it possible that all those who have murdered your and my people in your name have managed to reconcile their compassion toward you with a hatred for us? Has the institutionalization of humanity made humans inhuman? Has the universally accepted sorrow for your suffering provided the excuse to engage in cruelty to others without an afterthought?

No, I don't want to look at you. I would rather look at someone else, someone who could see you in millions of others, in ordinary, everyday people—one who could follow them to the ultimate border without turning away from them. Is it not him we are searching for in this century of Auschwitz and Hiroshima that is now approaching its end? Where can we find him? We search, but we do not find. We search and hope to find him in the fleeting figures who were with us for a little while and then vanished into the darkness without a trace. Raoul Wallenberg? Yes, exactly, and a few others. The towering symbol of compassion who was imprisoned and probably murdered without compassion. We turn our eyes away, we see but we don't see, we imagine that we might bring him back, but we know we cannot. We see, but we do not see.

Schopenhauer's "blind will," the urge for life that impels everything in the world, the innermost drive of all living organisms, is subdivided among an enormous number of individuals of each species. But this division, which Schopenhauer calls the "principle of individuation" (*principium individuationis*), does not weaken the will. On the contrary—the will is expressed with undiminished force in each organism. The will has no limits and no goal, it is an endless striving. The principle of individuation leads to competition among the members of each species for the resources of life. This strife manifests itself in humans with the most terrible clarity (*furchtbarste Deutlichkeit*). As a result, they can behave like wolves with one another (*homo homini lupus*).

In Schopenhauer's view, moral behavior can be based only on an intuitive recognition of your own self in every other human being. This attitude stems from an inner experience that cannot be taught through lectures or sermons. According to Schopenhauer, it is dangerous to base our most important concepts of life and our own role in the world on such ephemeral phenomena as dogmas, doctrines, or philosophical teachings.

Only a recognition of one's own being in others can generate *Mitleid*, or empathy, a word that Schopenhauer equates with *Liebe*, love, *agape, caritas, pietà*, and which he sees as the only pure form of love. Good deeds should not be driven by religious or ethical motives, to ensure a favorable place in heaven, or by the ambition to obtain rewards and recognition during earthly life. Such deeds are selfish and have no moral value. Schopenhauer even disapproves of the common concept of love built on mutual giving and receiving. Love can only come from "the knowledge of the suffering of others, which is directly understood when it is equated with your own suffering. It follows that pure love is the same as compassion, no matter whether it is directed toward great or small suffering." [5]

Here Schopenhauer distances himself from his esteemed colleague, "the great Kant," who recognizes true goodness and virtue only if it derives from abstract reflection and is based on the concepts of duty and the categorical imperative. To Kant, sympathy is not only not a virtue, but a weakness. No, says Schopenhauer, the concept of duty is equally foreign for true love as it is for true art. All true and pure love is compassion, and all love that is not compassion is selfishness. Schopenhauer admits that a combination of selfishness and empathy is closer to reality, and genuine friendship is always a mixture of the two. But he is adamant on his principle and he pursues the argument to its ultimate, logically consistent but absurd conclusion.

But one who has seen through the deception of the *principium individuationis*, and has succeeded in separating himself from it to such a degree that he can recognize himself, his innermost being, in all other beings, must be able to feel the endless suffering of all others and thereby experience the pain of the entire world. The sufferings of others are equally important to him as individual suffering is to the egoist. Schopenhauer concludes logically that relief can come only by turning away from life, by attaining a state of complete and perfect absence of the will. It is at this point that Schopenhauer changes from a rigorous, incisive, and almost modern analyst of the perpetual movements of biology to an ascetic prophet of resignation.

The first step in asceticism must be voluntary and total chastity, because sexuality is the highest manifestation of the blind, egoistic will. In ecstatic words reminiscent of religious texts, Schopenhauer extolls the virtues of self-denial and the constant struggle against the temptations of life that had been the earlier goals of all striving. Asceticism is sacred, death is deliverance. If one didn't know that these words were written by a great atheistic philosopher, one might easily believe that they come from a medieval theological text. But you only need to turn back one hundred pages in Schopenhauer's *The World as Will and Idea,* to his description of the world of biology, to get an entirely different impression. You may be tempted to replace the word "will" with "selfish gene" or "selfish DNA"[6] and come to the hasty conclusion that Schopenhauer understood the basic concepts of evolution half a century before Darwin and without any education in biology. But even if Schopenhauer wrote of biology and nature as if he were a biologist long before his time, he transforms paradoxically into a medieval philosopher when he refuses to accept the battle for existence and the perpetual struggle of the genes for survival as the most important principles of evolution. He commits a fundamental logical error when he disregards the fact that he could rise to the sublime and elevated spiritual vantage point of the philosopher only by using his brain, the most perfect accomplishment of evolution, or in his own words, of the blind will and its struggles. In contrast to his usual crystal-clear thinking, he shrinks from the obvious conclusion that the brain evolved originally as an instrument of battle in the same way as teeth, claws, and snake poison. By doing so, he makes his own position impossible and reaches an impasse—he wants to use the ultimate product of evolution, the brain, to halt evolution. He uses logic to reject the organic basis of all thinking, including logic itself. He even takes the wind out of the sails of his own wonderfully human and humane conclusion that equates empathy with love, and sets it as the highest goal of human spiritual development.

It is interesting to contrast Schopenhauer's reasoning with the thoughts of Nietzsche. These two among the greatest philosophers of the nineteenth century describe the world and humans in very similar terms, but they reach diametrically opposed conclusions. Early in his development, Nietzsche (1844–1900) followed Schopenhauer (1788–1868) and considered him one of his most important educators (*Erzieher*) and models. Around the same time, about 1868, his strong attachment to Schopenhauer's thinking was further reinforced by his great admiration for Wagner. In that year Wagner wrote *Die Meistersinger* and had long conversations with Nietzsche about Schopenhauer, whom Wagner regarded as the greatest philosopher and the only one to comprehend the essence of music. The twenty-four-year-old Nietzsche saw this as an important confirmation. In spite of his age, he was already an eminent authority on classical philology and philosophy. Although the teachings of Aristotle, Plato, and the other Greek philosophers were at the center of his interest, his passion for philosophy was sparked by Schopenhauer rather than the Greeks. Schopenhauer's clear, concise, and comprehensive writing style was unique among German philosophers and no doubt contributed to his special attraction for writers and artists throughout the ages. His reputation among professional philosophers, however, was much lower. They prefered their own specialist jargon, much less penetrable to outsiders.

Nietzsche's correspondence during his youth with his friend Erwin Rodhe (1870) reflects how aware he was of his own fragility and how much he feared failure, but it also shows his conviction in the importance of his mission. From the beginning, he was attracted by Schopenhauer's pessimism and fully agreed with his disdain for the matters of everyday life and for the narrow-mindedness of the bourgeois. A man of genius couldn't possibly socialize with them. He both needed and was condemned to solitude. Schopenhauer's inadequate contacts with the realities of human society and the practical difficulties that resulted from them—partly his own doing—must have been perceived by the young Nietzsche as a kind of confirmation. The basically tragic view of the human predicament was a starting point for both philosophers, but it led them to quite different conclusions. The very same insight that led to Schopenhauer's exhortation to deny the world and especially the will evoked ecstatic delight in Nietzsche. He embraced lust and the driving force of the instincts, he glorified the primeval Dionysian chaos, the basis of all creation. For Nietzsche, the world had only an aesthetic, but no moral justification. At this point, Nietzsche's philosophy is in line with Wagner's theory of music and the arts.

Nietzsche reacted with increasing fury against Schopenhauer's "hostility to life," his "morbid identification" with the sick and feeble. He suspected that Schopenhauer's moral system, especially his emphasis on empathy, arose from his own personal fear of suffering. To Nietzsche, self-pity appeared to be the most repellant failure of character, and he attacked it with all his might. He found the notion of compassion with the suffering of others equally repulsive. A preoccupation with the unsuccessful and the miserable can only increase suffering. It is a kind of nihilism that tramples on all the instincts that strive to save life and increase its value. Compassion negates life, as also shown by Schopenhauer's logically consistent denial of the instincts. Nietzsche clearly understood that biological evolution was based on selection, and he saw through the absurd logic that followed inevitably from Schopenhauer's reasoning.

But if Schopenhauer's analysis of the biological world and his humanistic concept of far-reaching empathy collide, the life-affirming reasoning of Nietzsche also leads to absurd consequences, but in a different way. A discussion of Nietzsche's paradoxical and highly controversial points of view, which have fascinated so many writers, is best introduced by some biographical data.

If Schopenhauer was afraid of a suffering that he had never been confronted with, Nietzsche knew much more about it from his own experience. After his appointment in 1869 to the chair of classical philology at the University of Basel at the unprecedentedly young age of twenty-five, even before he received his doctorate, the young Nietzsche suffered from serious afflictions. Only ten years later he was forced to retire from his position because of poor health. His great work, *Geburt der Tragödie* (*The Birth of Tragedy*) encountered a mixed reception. According to several critics, it had a scientifically weak foundation and the argumentation was too subjective. His students had abandoned him and, even long before his retirement, he had become disillusioned with academic life. Afflicted with poor health, he moved constantly between hotels, small rented rooms, and a variety of health resorts, as if he could outrun his symptoms. He suffered from frequent attacks of fever, coughing, diarrhea, vomiting, weakness, cramps, catarrh, listlessness, hemorrhoids, shingles, eye inflammations, and periods of severe anguish. He was treated with all available remedies, including leeches, blister-forming ointments, and a diet that at times consisted of only broth and tea. He took long walks, accompanied only by his thoughts. Sometimes he asked a friend or a hired secretary to record his dictations, but he gave that up soon because he became rapidly irritated at his aids.

He often sat in badly heated rooms, wrapped in sweaters. At other times he went on long and uncomfortable train trips to countries with warmer climates, where he was plagued by the heat and dust and his sensitive eyes became irritated by the sun. His friends found it increasingly difficult to witness his suffering and gradually abandoned him. His relatively few enthusiastic readers stopped writing to him. In his deepening solitude Nietzsche wrote as if he were conducting a monologue with himself, which was simultaneously being heard by millions. In brilliant and often moving prose, he praised the triumph of strength, glorified violence in its many forms, and admired physical and mental power. An elite of "great men" are destined to rule the world. Only the "higher individual" the hero, the tyrannical ruler had a "high value." Human society and the entire history of the species can be justified only by having produced such great men. The suffering of the masses mattered but little compared to the struggles of these great men. The sole justification of the French Revolution was the fact that it permitted Napoleon's rise to power. "The revolution made Napoleon possible. That is its justification. For a similar price, one would welcome the total collapse of our entire civilization into anarchy. Napoleon made nationalism possible: that is its excuse."

Nietzsche's ruling elite were to be brought up in hardship and suffering. They must learn to endure abandonment, disease, maltreatment, and humiliation. They had to face the suffering of self-contempt and despair, but they had to rise above their own misery. "I have no compassion with them. I wish them the only possible proof of human value today—the ability to endure."

Nietzsche decided to reject Schopenhauer just at a time when Schopenhauer's pessimism had been of greater use to him than anything else. He continued writing while his eyesight was becoming so poor that he could hardly see what he had written, and even at times when his headaches were so severe that he could no longer hear his own thoughts. Is it possible that his hard attitude toward suffering and those who suffered was an expression of his absolute determination to stifle the slightest tendencies toward self-pity? Is this why he regarded the conquest of compassion as the greatest virtue? Is it one of the explanations of his aversion toward all forms of democratic reasoning? Is this why he spoke so contemptuously about the shepherd mentality that strives for the same green pastures for all, a concept that prevents the more highly creative person from improving the quality of life and of the species? How did he reconcile the hard struggle for self-control with other motivations that stemmed from his unique background, and particularly from his early rebellion against a dogmatic, narrow, and traditional upbringing that he countered with his own original, liberated perspectives? The tension between the Apollonian personality—to use Nietzsche's own expression—who loved the intoxication and exhilaration of Dionysus and the desperation of hopeless love must have been combined with his rebellion against his own suffering. Together they created the immense, primal power of his poetry, his ability to say yes when all others said no and to say no when all others said yes, his contemptuous criticism of the weak and lowly as we all are, and his fervent admiration of all that we could become if we could implement what he considered our hightest aspirations.

The reader of today who is not entranced by the charismatic language will have some difficulty accepting Nietzsche's total contempt for morality. He viewed it as the destroyer of all positive human qualities. There is no such thing as true morality. The so-called moral behavior of man stems neither from his unselfishness nor his goodwill, but is determined by external factors such as rewards and punishments. "Unselfishness" or altruism merely reflects an adaptation, a training of the individual to conform, to follow the herd. Although Nietzsche admitted that a morality based on this kind of adaptation can play an important role in real life, he dismissed the notion that man might transcend the trivial problems of existence and reach a higher plane of altruism and morality. This idea, he thought, is nothing but an illusion that can help man live, or masked egoism. In reality, all man's actions are motivated by "the urge for power." Truly altruistic actions are impossible. Claims to the contrary are nothing but fraudulent rhetoric and an abominable misrepresentation of human psychology. The average person, the herd creature, uses such rhetoric to conceal his own mediocrity, timidity, and weariness with life and with himself. It is part of his attempt to appear more noble, more important, more respectable, and more divine than he is, to reap more of the available benefits. The driving forces of morality meet its principles in a head-on collision.

Few who read Nietzsche can escape a certain fascination with his intellectual clarity, his remarkable prose, and by at least some of his vision. He continues to attract devoted followers in broad circles and sometimes in places where one would least expect them. Is this also due, at least in some small part, to the feelings elicited by his tragic fate? The road of the ailing genius from a brilliant youthful career to solitude, illness, and the final mental disintegration caused by progressive paralysis—the devastating last stage of tertiary syphilis that made him into an idiot, playing with dolls—is an image that readily awakens a feeling of combined respect and sympathy (*Ehrfurcht und Erbarmen*), as Thomas Mann expressed it.[7] There has been no lack of modern defenders of Nietzsche who have tried to soften some of his statements that were exploited and distorted by the Nazis half a century later. They have called attention to Nietzsche's disgust for governments and suggested that he would have become a radical foe of Nazism. They have also pointed out that Nietzsche was not anti-Semitic— he was in fact just the opposite. It has been shown that some of the letters found after his death were forged by his sister Elisabeth Förster, who was married to a notorious anti-Semite and who later became Hitler's personal friend. But what can one say about Nietzsche's *Götzendämmerung* (*Twilight of the Idols*), in which he praises the Indian "law of Manu" with its unrelenting caste system and its explicit instructions on the elimination of the lowly "raceless, hodgepodge creatures" (*Nicht-Zucht-Menschen, Mischmasch-Menschen*), the Chandala. According to the "law of Manu," one should strive to weaken the Chandala, to make them sick, to reduce their reproduction. Nietzsche comments, "One draws a breath of relief when coming out of the Christian hospital and dungeon atmosphere into this healthier, higher, *wider* world. How paltry the 'New Testament' is compared with Manu, how ill it smells!"[8]

The law of Chandala states further that untouchables are allowed to eat only unclean vegetables, to drink water only from the entrances to swamps and from holes made by the feet of animals—never from clean springs. They are also forbidden to wash themselves or their clothes, they are not to be given assistance during childbirth, and they should be exposed to all imaginable epidemics. "They shall have for clothing only rags from corpses, for utensils broken pots, for worship only evil spirits."

Nietzsche continues:

These regulations are instructive enough: in them, we find for once Aryan humanity, quite pure, quite primordial—we learn that the concept "pure blood" is not a harmless concept. It becomes clear how the Chandala hatred has been mobilized against this form of "humanity," how it has been made into a religion. The Gospels are the most important documents from this point of view. Christianity, growing from Jewish roots and comprehensible only as a product of this soil, represents the reaction against that morality of breeding, of race, of privilege—it is the *anti-Aryan* religion *par excellence.* Christianity is the reevaluation of all Aryan values, the victory of Chandala values, the evangel preached to the poor and lowly, the collective rebellion of everything downtrodden, wretched, ill-constituted, under-privileged against the "race"—undying Chandala revenge as the *religion of love.*[9]

I was trying to find some excuse for these words. I hoped that they might have originated from the forgeries of Nietzsche's sister. Experts on Nietzsche have assured me, however, that the text is authentic, but it was written only a couple of years before his mental breakdown.[10]

Although I have tried very hard, I could finally not avoid seeing the horrible similiarity of these words to the speech by the mass murderer Heinrich Himmler on October 4, 1943. He made it perfectly clear that Nazism was about to destroy "the Jewish race" that he regarded as vermin. He praised the members of the SS who were able to look at hundreds or even thousands of dead bodies and yet remain "decent people." "This is a glorious part of our history that has never been and will never be written" (*ein niemals geschriebenes und niemals zu schreibendes Ruhmesblatt*), he continued. "We have the moral right, it is our duty to our nation to destroy these people who wanted to destroy us."[11]

Nietzsche was an extraordinary writer and a great philosopher. Himmler was the worst mass murderer in the history of the world, unless you want to save this title for his Führer. I would prefer not to write the names Himmler and Nietzsche on the same piece of paper. But my hand moves inexorably and I cannot find any more compelling argument against it than my own discomfort. That is not enough to stay my hand.

I feel an almost uncontrollable wish to forgive that sick, desperate philosopher who longed so fervently for a nobler life, but who projected his own suffering and his merciless self-flagellation as if they would apply to all of humanity, of which he only saw a very limited part. But no forgiveness should ever be extended to the mass murderer who performed his deeds brutally and coldly, sparing not children, women, or the elderly. Over the accursed memory of Himmler, I would like to read the words of Moses, as spoken by Thomas Mann in *Das Gesetz* (*The Tables of the Law*), written in 1943. I will never forget the moment in 1944 when I was in a cellar in German-occupied Budapest, listening illegally to Thomas Mann himself reading from his book over the BBC's German-language program.

Thus speaks God to Moses about the man who will break his commandments that were given on Mount Sinai shortly before: *"In den Erdengrund will Ich den Lästerer treten hundert und zwölf Klafter tief, und Mensch und Tier sollen einen Bogen machen um die Stätte wo Ich ihn hineintrat, und die Vögel des Himmels hoch im Fluge ausweichen, dass sie nicht darüber fliegen. Und wer seinen Namen nennt, der soll nach allen vier Gegenden speien und sich den Mund wischen und sprechen: 'Behüte!'"* ("To the bottom of the earth I will tread the blasphemer, an hundred and twelve fathoms deep, and man and beast shall make a bend around the spot where I trod him in, and the birds of the air high in their flight shall swerve that they fly not over it. And whosoever names his name shall spit towards the four quarters of the earth, and wipe his mouth and say 'God save us all!'")

Sils-Maria, 1985

I am standing in Nietzsche's bedroom. How small it is! What a narrow, short little bed, what a tiny washbasin! Nietzsche's cave (*Höhle*), as he called it, referring to Zarathustra, was on the top floor of a plain farmhouse, only a few steps from the main road. He rented it for one franc per day. His childhood friend and newly appointed professor of philosophy Paul Deussen described the interior of the rooms: "Some bookcases, a simple table with a coffee pot, eggshells, manuscripts, toilet articles in a mess, boots fallen over on the floor, an unmade bed."[12]

It was here, then, where he sat and wrote, where he had his migraine attacks, where his unique brain, undermined by an accidentally and senselessly acquired infection during his youth, darkened gradually on the way to the inevitable collapse. The master of the German language and its greatest poet in prose, the angriest prophet of the last century wrote *Also sprach Zarathustra* (*Thus Spake Zarathustra—A Book for All and None*) in this little room!

It is getting dark. I follow the path around the peninsula that juts out into the shimmering lake, one of his favorite walks. A large inscribed stone has been erected at the outermost point. From it I read "Das trunkene Lied" from *Zarathustra*, a poem I used to know by heart:

Oh. Mensch! Gib Acht!
Was spricht die tiefe Mitternacht?
Ich schlief, ich schlief—
Aus tiefem Traum bin ich erwacht:—
Die Welt ist tief,
Und tiefer als der Tag gedacht.
Tief ist ihr Weh—
Lust tiefer noch als Herzeleid:
Weh spricht: Vergeh!
Doch alle Lust will Ewigkeit—
—Will tiefe, tiefe Ewigkeit! [13]

O man, take care!
What does the deep midnight declare?
"I was asleep—
From a deep dream I woke and swear:
The world is deep,
Deeper than day had been aware.
Deep is its woe;
Joy—deeper yet than agony:
Woe implores: Go!
But all joy wants eternity—
Wants deep, wants deep eternity."

All joy wants eternity. What does that mean? The pleasure of orgasm and its biological goal, the perpetuation of the species? Or the pleasure of the soul, the exhilaration of creativity that he wished to protect from the increasingly colorless commercialized pseudoculture of the masses? The joy of the romantic hero, or the pleasure of the powerful elite built on slavery, oppression, torture, and murder? All and none of these?

Schopenhauer and Nietzsche have passed on to eternity, but we are left with their dilemma. Their almost identical analysis of the inherent tragedy of life is as relevant today as it was in their time. We can look at their diametrically opposed conclusions with the same amazement as their contemporary readers, but from the vantage point of a wider and more bitter experience. Shortly after the Second World War, one of the most knowledgeable observers took a fresh look at Nietzsche's work.[14] In a speech delivered in 1947, Thomas Mann examined Nietzsche's thesis that there is no authority in front of which "life" should be ashamed of anything at all. Thomas Mann questions this conclusion. Even if we would ignore the question of morality, as Nietzsche wants us to do, we have every reason to reflect over spirituality, humanity, and the resulting judgments, as they are expressed in criticism and irony, and as they manifest themselves in a concept of human freedom. Spirituality is the self-criticism of life; it permits nature and life to transcend themselves. Thomas Mann views Nietzsche's "teaching of health" with a mixture of skepticism and compassion. After having started his career as a critic of true "historical illness," Nietzsche has come to angrily reject everything that could tame the wild life, including all morality, religion, and humanism. Mann identifies two basic flaws in Nietzsche's thinking. One is his misjudgment of the power balance between the instincts and the intellect. Nietzsche sees the intellect as the principal threat, from whose domination the instincts must be rescued. But in reality the instincts—or rather the will, the term that both Schopenhauer and Nietzsche used—are dominant over both reason and justice. Should the defeat of the intellect require the assistance of the instinct? "As if there is even the slightest chance that the intellect could ever get the upper hand here on earth!" Mann commented only two years after Hitler had disappeared from the world scene. On the contrary, there is every reason to protect the flickering flames of decency, intellect, and justice rather than stand on the side of power and instinct, whose horrible insanity we have recently experienced. There is no risk at all that culture would destroy life. "Life is a tough cat and so is mankind."

According to Thomas Mann, Nietzsche commits his second serious mistake when he views life and morality as antagonists. On the contrary—they belong together. The true conflict is between ethics and aesthetics. It is not morality, but the "beauty" as worshipped by Nietzsche and, among others, Oscar Wilde, that is doomed. Many poets have spoken about this—wouldn't Nietzsche have known about it? Ethics and morality support life; the ethical person is its true pillar, possibly somewhat uninteresting but very useful. Nietzsche commented contemptuously that Socrates and

Plato ceased being true Greeks and became Jews when they began speaking of truth and justice. At this point, one can almost see Thomas Mann shaking his head with the good-natured but nevertheless mercilessly incisive sarcasm that characterizes all of his work, especially his four Joseph novels. "Thanks to their sense of morality, the Jews have proven to be the good and perseverant children of life. They have survived the millennia while the small groups of aesthetic and artistic peoples such as the Greeks have rapidly vanished from the historical scene."

Thomas Mann also points out that Nietzsche did not display the slightest trace of anti-Semitism. Rather, he rejected everything that he saw as the morality of a "flock of sheep," which included, in his view, "all sorts of shopkeepers and merchants, Christians, cows, women, Englishmen, and other democrats." He praises the tradition of human sacrifice and claims that Christianity put an end to natural selection. He extols the rights of strong men to sacrifice the weak, millions if necessary, to promote the supermen of the future. Thomas Mann asked, who has espoused this idea during this century, who have so arrogantly granted themselves this power? A petty gang of megalomaniacal bourgeois in whose presence Nietzsche would have immediately been struck by a severe migraine attack.

But even if the humanist Thomas Mann condemns Nietzsche's ideas in his uncompromising, slightly satirical, and yet respectful way, what are the views of the biologists and geneticists? After all, Nietzsche's disagreement with Schopenhauer had a "biological" basis. He could not accept that Schopenhauer shrank from the cruelty of nature, the power of blind will, the instincts, the ravages of competition, struggles, and war, and chose to withdraw into the nirvana of asceticism and seclusion. Nietzsche saw clearly that this seemingly impressive aesthetic position was a senseless revolt of the soul against the body whose product it was and that this would lead to an impasse, the suicide of the species. "Above all, we must renounce Schopenhauer," he writes in *Götzendämmerung*. Nietzsche's own glorification of the "superman" seems to have a biological basis, but its biology is perverted. The greatest "hero" of evolution is not he who kills the greatest number of foes. It is not Siegfried with his sword "Notung," sailing joyfully down the Rhine after having slain the dragon. The real hero is the one who succeeds in passing on his genetic material to the greatest number of children. One of this century's greatest geneticists, Theodosius Dobzhansky, has expressed it in the following way:

The survival of the fittest does not mean that just one fittest variant survives and the rest die: what is fit to survive, survives. . . . In vain did some naturalists point out that success in the struggle for existence is at least as often achieved among animals by cooperation and mutual help as by competition and combat. Many people prefer to take Darwin's metaphors quite literally. The idea that struggle without quarter or mercy is a universal law of Nature and that harsh and ruthless competition results in biological progress and improvement were grasped as ready justifications of power politics, conquest, exploitation of the weak by the strong, child labor and even laissez-faire economics. Racism, which reached its ugliest forms in Hitler's Germany but which is still very much alive in South Africa and in many places closer to home, also tries to appear decent and "scientific" in a Darwinian garb.

Such attempts to misuse the theory of evolution as an excuse for man's inhumanity to man are evidently a travesty of science. Not all is sweetness and light in biological nature. . . . But it does not follow that humans must stalk, strangulate and devour each other. . . . The development of genetics has made possible a better understanding of natural selection. The selectively fit or, if you will, the fittest, is not necessarily a fellow with big muscles or a lusty fighter, or a conqueror of all his competitors. He is, rather, a paterfamilias who has raised a large number of children who in turn become patres familias. . . . Darwinian fitness is reproductive fitness.[15]

One might possibly object that Dobzhansky's arguments are apologetic and somewhat artificial from a purely biological point of view. But in the final analysis, the biological discussion is irrelevant. The central argument is based on the ethically and morally determined concept that all humans have equal rights and that injustice and slavery are abominable. These are humane and humanitarian values that are, and must remain, independent of all evolutionary considerations. There is a central logical flaw in comparisons of Nietzsche and Darwin. Darwin was a natural scientist. His goal was to describe nature as it appeared to him. The ideological extrapolator is always responsible for his extrapolation—this is not the province of the biologist. Philosophers like Nietzsche have a completely different goal. They want to teach us how life should be lived. They are therefore fully responsible for the consequences of their concepts, even if they have made a large number of disparate statements, endorsing opposing positions in different writings. That was certainly true of Nietzsche. There are many discussions today on the responsibility of the scientist, even in cases when it is obvious that the negative effects of a certain scientific discovery stemmed from political applications or distortions of science, rather than from science itself. The philosopher has a more immediate responsibility, because he can influence the ethical and moral values of his audience to a much greater extent.

The perversion of Nietzsche's philosophy and the pseudo-aesthetics, dehumanization, and apocalyptic nihilism of Nazism has, once and for all, put an end to the myth of the romantic hero, or so one would like to hope. The two great philosophers, Nietzsche and Schopenhauer, have therefore neutralized each other, in a way. For me, Schopenhauer's concept of *Mitleid*, the compassion that can arise from insight about the illusory nature of the individuation principle and from the resulting identification with every other member of the human species, remains one of the most beautiful thoughts ever conceived. But my own Mitleid has its limits. I do want to include Nietzsche—the sick, condemned, and lost philosopher who fought so ardently against the idea, possibly to avert the self-pity that he had so much reason to feel. But it does reject those who chose to put Nietzsche's ideas into practice during the even more pathological century that followed.

Darkness has now almost completely closed in over the lake. Here Nietzsche stood, in the shadows of the great mountains, dreaming of the superman who could overcome his human weaknesses even as the inexorable darkness came upon him and extinguished his shining vision of the future. This modern prophet, whose words will endure forever through the primal voice of his poetry, despite its frequently repulsive content, was already beginning to transform into a living corpse destined to vegetate for another eleven meaningless years. I am overwhelmed by the compassion that he so fervently disdained. Or did he really? His final collapse came on January 3, 1889, at the Piazza Carlo Alberto in Turin, after many warning signals, rapidly deteriorating contact with reality, and an increasing megalomania. He had just come out of his apartment when he saw a coach driver brutally mistreating his horse. Plaintively objecting, he threw himself over the horse, embracing it around the neck, and collapsed.

I feel the same pietà that Schopenhauer equates with love. Helplessly and against all better judgment, I know that I love that wonderful, dreadful, and desperate genius who, like Zarathustra, *"verliess seine Höhle, glühend und stark wie eine Morgensonne, die aus dunklen Bergen kommt"* (left his cave, glowing and strong as a morning sun that comes out of dark mountains).[15]

Notes

Introduction

1. Albert Camus, *The Myth of Sisyphus, and Other Essays,* translated by Justin O'Brien. New York: Alfred A. Knopf, 1958.

2. *The Divine Comedy of Dante Alighieri,* translated by A. Mandelbaum. Toronto: Bantam Books, 1984.

3. Ibid.

4. Arthur Schopenhauer, *The World as Will and Idea,* translated by R. B. Haldane and J. Kemp. London: Routledge & Kegan Paul, 1964.

Part Two: Suicides

Translator's note: The word "suicide" is derived from the Latin *sui,* meaning "of oneself" and *cidium,* from *caedere,* meaning "to kill." It therefore means voluntary "self-killing," a phrase close to the word "self-killer" that the author equates with the Swedish *självmördare* for "suicide."

Pista

1. Charles Baudelaire, "The Voyage," from Book III, *The Flowers of Evil,* translated by P. J. W. Higson and E. R. Ashe. Chester: Cestrian Press, 1975.

2. The name Pista should be pronounced "Pishta." It is a diminutive form of István, equivalent to Stephen.

Attila József

1. *Attila József Poems,* edited by T. Kabdebo. Poem translated by Thomas Kabdebo. London: The Danubia Book Co., 1966.

2. Arthur Koestler, *The Invisible Writing—An Autobiography.* New York: MacMillan, 1954.

3. *Attila József: Selected Poems and Texts,* edited by G. Gömöri and J. Atlas, translated by J. Bátki. Iowa City, Iowa: International Writing Program.

4. *Nyugat* (*The West*) was the most distinguished Hungarian literary magazine, in which the works of the most important poets of the time were published. These included Endre Ady, Babits, and Kosztolányi. The name of the magazine was a clear indication of the tendency of the new Hungarian poetry to break with the romantic nationalistic Hungarian tradition and establish ties with the poetry of Western Europe.

5. Koestler, *Invisible Writing.*

6. *Poems of Attila József,* edited by Joseph M. Értavy-Baráth, translated by Anton N. Nyerges. New York: Hungarian Cultural Foundation, 1973.

7. From *Perched on Nothing's Branch: Selected Poetry of Attila Jósef,* translated by Peter Hargitai. Tallahassee, FL: Apalachee Press, 1987.

8. A. Bókay, F. Jádi, and A. Stark, *Köztelek lettem én bolond.* Budapest, 1982.

9. *Attila József: Selected Poems and Texts.*

10. Ibid.

11. *Attila József Poems.* Poem translated by M. Hamburger.

12. *Poems of Attila József.*

13. Poem translated by T. Kabdebo.

14. *Kalevala,* compiled by E. Lönnrot, translated by W.F. Kirby, Runo XVII, pp. 248-250. London: J.M.Dent and Sons, 1907.

15. J. Szántó, *Napló és visszaemlékezés (Diary and Memories).* Budapest, 1986.

16. Bókay, Jádi, and Stark, *Köztelek lettern én bolond.*

17. *Poems of Attila József.*

18. Ibid.

19. Ibid.

20. *Attila József: Selected Poems and Texts.*

21. *Poems of Attila József.*

22. Illyés Gyuláne, *József Attila utolsó hónapjairól (József Attila's Last Months).* Budapest, 1987.

23. *Attila József Poems.* Poem translated by T. Kabdebo.

24. *Attila József Poems.* Poem translated by Vernon Watkins.

25. *Poems of Attila József.*

26. Márta Vágó, *József Attila.* Budapest, 1975.

27. *Hungarian Anthology. A collection of poems,* translated by J. Grosz and W. A. Boggs. Toronto: Pannonia Books, 1966.

28. *Attila József Poems.* Poem translated by Vernon Watkins.

29. Bertalan Hatvany was an orientalist, aristocrat, and Attila's close friend and patron.

Orpheus

1. *Kalevala*, compiled by E. Lönnrot, translated by W. F. Kirby, Runo XLIV. London: J. M. Dent and Sons, 1907.

2. C. J. Burckhart, *Ein Vormittag beim Buchhändler*. Basel, 1945.

3. Rainer Maria Rilke, *The Book of Hours*. New Directions, 1941.

4. *The Selected Poetry of Rainer Maria Rilke*, edited and translated by S. Mitchell. New York: Vintage International Books, 1980.

5. Libretto to *Orpheus* by C. von Gluck, translated by Rev. J. Troutbeck. London: Novello and Co., 1951.

6. *Kalevala*, Runo III.

7. Ibid., Runo XL.

8. Ibid.

9. Ibid.

10. Ibid., Runo XLI.

11. Ibid.

12. Edgar Allan Poe, "Ulalume," in *Complete Stories and Poems of Edgar Allan Poe*. Garden Grove, N.Y.: Doubleday & Co., 1966.

13. *Edgar Allan Poe: Selected Prose and Poetry*, edited by W. H. Auden. New York, 1962.

The Ultimate Fear of the Traveler Returning from Hell

1. R. Vrba and A. Bestic, *I Cannot Forgive*. 1964.

2. M. Gilbert, *Auschwitz and the Allies*. New York, 1981.

3. George Mikes, *Sunday Times*, February 2, 1964.

4. Miklós Nyiszli, *Auschwitz. An Eyewitness Report*. New York, 1960.

5. B. Müller-Hill, *Murderous Science*. Oxford: Oxford University Press, 1988. See also the chapter "Ultima Thule," in George Klein, *The Atheist and the Holy City*, translated by Theodore and Ingrid Friedmann. Cambridge, MA: MIT Press, 1990.

6. M. Gilbert, *The Holocaust*. New York, 1985.

7. Vrba referred to a statement by General Rudolf Hoffmann, commander of the northern army, as quoted by H. A. Jacobsen and J. Rohwer in *Decisive Battles of World War II: The German View*. London, 1966.

8. H. Langbein, *Wir haben es gesehen*. Vienna, 1964.

9. Robert J. Lifton, *The Nazi Doctors*. New York, 1986.

10. Bruno Bettelheim, *Surviving and Other Essays*. New York, 1952.

11. "Erinnerungen an Julius Hallervorden, 1882–1965," in *Der Nervenarzt*, 1966.

12. Müller-Hill, *Murderous Science.*

13. Nyiszli, *Auschwitz. An Eyewitness Report.*

The Fatherless

1. Jean-Paul Sartre, *The Words,* translated by Bernard Frechtman. New York: Vintage Books, 1964.

2. The phrase "Jante law" refers to the Swedish aphorism, "You must not believe that you are a somebody" (*Du skall icke tro att du är någon*). The phrase is used as a kind of warning from one Swede to another not to stand out too much from the crowd. It is often typical of the attitude of bureaucrats and authorities toward people of distinction.

3. D. K. Simonton, *Scientific Genius.* Cambridge, 1988.

4. C. Martindale, *Psychological Reports* 31 (1972): 843–847.

5. Walberg et al., *Journal of Creative Behaviour* 13 (1980): 225–231.

6. G. C. Zahn, *In Solitary Witness: The Life and Death of Franz Jägerstätter.* New York: Holt, Rinehart and Winston, 1964.

6. Ibid.

Biological Individuality

1. R.P. De Vries, P. Meera Khan, L. F. Bernini, E. van Loghen, and J. J. van Rood, "Genetic control of survival in epidemics," *Journal of Immunogenetics* 6(1979): 271–287.

2. Osoba et al., *Journal of Immunogenetics* 8(1979): 323.

3. Geczy et al., *Annals of Rheumatic Diseases* 46(1987): 171.

4. George Klein, *The Atheist and the Holy City.*

5. Ibid.

AIDS

1. K. K. Holmes, and J. Kreis, "Heterosexual transmission of HIV: Overview of a neglected aspect of the AIDS epidemic," *Journal of AIDS* 1(1988): 602–661.

2. J. H. Gagnon, "Sex research and sexual conduct in the era of AIDS," *Journal of AIDS* 1 (1988): 593–601.

3. George Klein, "Coexistence between Virus and Man," in *The Atheist and the Holy City.*

4. Klein, "Viruses and Cancer," in *The Atheist and the Holy City.*

5. Ibid.

6. Klein, "Blind Will and Selfish DNA," in *The Atheist and the Holy City.*

7. Klein, "Coexistence between Virus and Man."

8. Klein, "Peter Noll's Awareness of Death and Wisdom of Life," in *The Atheist and the Holy City.*

9. Peter Noll, *In the Face of Death.* Viking Press, 1989.

Pietà

1. Rainer Maria Rilke, *Alcestis,* from *Rainer Maria Rilke, Selected Works,* translated by J.B. Leishman. Norfolk: Hogarth Press, 1960.

2. Lamentationes I.12 Nova Vulgata Bibliorum Sacrorum. Libreria Editrice Vaticana, 1979.

3. Rainer Maria Rilke, untitled poem from *The Book of Hours,* Third Book, in *Selected Works,* vol. II, translated by J. B. Leishman. Norfolk: Hogarth Press, 1960. I urge readers to read Rilke's wonderful poem first in the German if possible, even if it is difficult. If you must read the translation, go back to the German afterward—it is worth the trouble.

4. Marguerite Duras, *Hiroshima Mon Amour,* translated by R.Seaver. New York: Grove Press, 1961.

5. Arthur Schopenhauer, *The World as Will and Idea* translated by R. B. Haldane and J. Kemp. London: Routledge & Kegan Paul, 1964, p. 485.

6. In my earlier book, *The Atheist and the Holy City,* I discussed the similarities between Schopenhauer's *will* and the modern view of selfish DNA in the chapter "Blind Will and Selfish DNA."

7. Thomas Mann, *Nietzsche's Philosophie im Lichte unserer Erfahrung,* 1947. Frankfurt, 1982.

8. F. Nietzsche, *Twilight of the Idols,* translated by R.J. Hollingdale. London: Penguin Books, 1968.

9. Ibid.

10. For further discussions concerning the significance of this text of the Nazi ideology, see Benno Müller-Hill, "Die Wissenschaft von der biologischen Auslese von Uenschen." In *Medizin und Gesundheitspolitik der NS-Zeit,* edited by N. Frei, 1990.

11. M. Gilbert, *The Holocaust.* New York, 1985.

12. This description and other biographical notes are taken from I. Frenzel, *Friedrich Nietzsche,* Hamburg, 1966.

13. F. Nietzsche, *Thus Spoke Zarathustra,* translated by Walter Kaufmann. London: Penguin Books, 1954.

14. Mann, *Nietzsche's Philosophie im Lichte unserer Erfahrung.*

15. T. Dobzhansky, *Heredity and the Nature of Man.* New York: Harcourt, Brace and World, 1964.

16. Nietzsche, *Thus Spoke Zarathustra.*

Index